Cancer: A Very Short Introduction

VERY SHORT INTRODUCTIONS are for anyone wanting a stimulating and accessible way into a new subject. They are written by experts, and have been translated into more than 45 different languages.

The series began in 1995, and now covers a wide variety of topics in every discipline. The VSI library now contains over 500 volumes—a Very Short Introduction to everything from Psychology and Philosophy of Science to American History and Relativity—and continues to grow in every subject area.

Titles in the series include the following:

Nicholas James

CANCER

A Very Short Introduction

OXFORD
UNIVERSITY PRESS

OXFORD

UNIVERSITY PRESS

Great Clarendon Street, Oxford OX2 6DP

Oxford University Press is a department of the University of Oxford.
It furthers the University's objective of excellence in research, scholarship,
and education by publishing worldwide in

Oxford New York

Auckland Cape Town Dar es Salaam Hong Kong Karachi
Kuala Lumpur Madrid Melbourne Mexico City Nairobi
New Delhi Shanghai Taipei Toronto

With offices in

Argentina Austria Brazil Chile Czech Republic France Greece
Guatemala Hungary Italy Japan Poland Portugal Singapore
South Korea Switzerland Thailand Turkey Ukraine Vietnam

Oxford is a registered trade mark of Oxford University Press
in the UK and in certain other countries

Published in the United States
by Oxford University Press Inc., New York

© Nicholas James 2011

British Library Cataloguing in Publication Data
Data available

Library of Congress Cataloging in Publication Data
Data available

Typeset by SPI Publisher Services, Pondicherry, India

Printed and bound by
CPI Group (UK) Ltd, Croydon, CR0 4YY

ISBN: 978-0-19-956023-3

Contents

Acknowledgements

Writing even a small book such as this is a big undertaking. I'd like to acknowledge the help and support given by my wife Alison and by my family in giving me the time and space needed to produce this book. I'd also like to thank my parents for the massive contributions they made to supporting my education, often at great personal sacrifice.

List of illustrations

Chapter 1
The size of the cancer problem

Cancer is common, very common. In 2008, around 12.7 million people were diagnosed with cancer, of whom 7.9 million died, accounting for around 13% of all deaths. Although there is a perception that cancer is a disease of the aged population in the richer economies, around 70% of these deaths occurred in low- or middle-income countries. Cancer affects both genders, all races, rich and poor alike. The diagnosis is feared, as it is assumed (often correctly) to be a death sentence by those afflicted with it. Both the disease itself and its treatment are major causes of pain and distress. Treating cancer is a major burden on healthcare systems worldwide, and the disease is a significant cause of loss of productive capacity within the workforce due to premature death. This chapter will take an overview of the cancer problem, focusing on some of the more common cancers to illustrate how numbers vary across the world. Any illness affecting so many people will also have major economic impacts, so this chapter will also highlight some of the ways in which the economy and health services interact, themes that will be developed further in later chapters. Studying patterns in rates of cancer sheds very interesting light on the causes of cancer (covered more fully in Chapter 2). Some of the most striking links will be highlighted in this chapter as well.

Cancer care and cancer research are also important components of industrial activity. Half of all drugs in clinical trials are for cancer; the global market for all cancer drugs was estimated at $48 billion in 2008, up from $34.6 billion in 2006. Analysts expect growth from 2010 to 2015 to be above 10% annually. Every year, the pharmaceutical industry spends between $6.5 and $8 billion on research and development of cancer drugs. This spend dwarfs that from government and research charities on drug development, potentially meaning that new drugs are concentrated in areas with maximum commercial rather than public health impact. Pharmaceutical companies with successful cancer drugs are among the biggest corporations worldwide. Biotech companies without marketable products but with a promising 'pipeline' cancer drug can be worth billions of dollars simply because of the possibility that the drug may be licensed at some future date for treating cancer. At least 19 anticancer drugs exceeded $1 billion in sales in 2009, a major strain for health systems in even the richest economies charged with purchasing these drugs for their patients.

At the other end of the spectrum, around one-third of cancer patients have very limited access to effective treatments, rising to over half in the poorest countries. Moving forwards, with an ageing population and rising drug price trends, we may get to the situation when 'state-of-the-art' drug therapy will be available only to the richest strata in the richest economies. Alternatively, better prediction of response to therapy may allow individually targeted treatment choices, reducing costs from unnecessary or ineffective therapy. Unlike, say, cars or computers, which we expect to work every time we use them, most cancer drugs work on only a proportion of patients. For those with advanced disease, for whom the aim is palliation of symptoms or improvement in quality of life, this proportion may be much less than 50%, hence the majority of treatments may be pointless, or indeed worse than useless, as they may cause side effects with no benefit. Being able to identify patients who may benefit ahead of therapy would be very cost and clinically effective and this is therefore a major focus of current cancer research (see Chapters 4 and 5).

Cancer has also fascinated the world's academics and universities. In 1961, John F. Kennedy pledged to put a man on the moon by the end of the decade. Nine years later, Neil Armstrong and Buzz Aldrin walked on the moon. Ten years later, in 1971, Richard Nixon echoed this pledge by declaring a 'war' on cancer. Rather like the more recent 'war on terror', picking a fight with a multifaceted worldwide problem has been at best only partly successful. Nixon's initial pledge was around $100 million, which seemed like a bonanza at the time, but has turned out to barely scratch the surface. Since 1971, billions more research dollars have followed, but more than 30 years later cancer remains one of the largest causes of death worldwide, with around 1 in 3 developing the disease in developed economies and 1 in 5 in the West dying from it. Curing cancer is clearly harder than 'rocket science'.

Worldwide, huge amounts are spent on research into the causes and treatment of cancer. In 2009/10, the US National Cancer Institute spent $4.7 billion on cancer research; equivalent spend in Europe was around €1.4 billion. In the UK, the biggest spender is Cancer Research UK, one of the largest British charities, which in 2010 had an annual income from donations of more than £500 million, reflecting the importance attached to finding causes and cures for cancer among the wider population (the foremost recipients of public donations are, however, animals not people!). Despite this vast expenditure on research, we still do not really understand what causes a substantial proportion of cancers. Furthermore, despite the money spent on drugs and drug research, for the majority of patients cured of cancer, this is as a result of either surgery or radiotherapy, as described in Chapter 3. Chemotherapy and other newer treatments such as monoclonal antibodies or targeted 'small molecule' therapies, while growing in importance, still account for only a minority of cures but have a major role in palliation of advanced disease symptoms.

There are various ways of looking at the problem cancer poses. These range from the raw numbers – how many people diagnosed, how many people die – to the personal – what is your individual risk of getting a particular cancer? Population-based statistics can be presented in various ways, from rates for the whole population to rates adjusted by age to calculations on numbers of years of life lost. These latter statistics are often expressed as years lost before the age of 70 – the biblical 'three score years and ten' – thereby assuming that deaths after 70 (or sometimes 75) essentially represent death from old age. A further complication is that deaths from cancer vary enormously by income, race, and country of residence. For example, breast and prostate cancers are much more common in Europe and North America than in Japan and China. Migrants from these countries to the United States progressively alter their risk of these cancers towards that of white Americans but retain a lower overall risk. This tells us that the lower rates of breast and prostate cancer in the Far East are partly down to environment and partly down to racial differences or some linked aspect of the environment that is portable – diet, for example.

To try and explore these concepts further, I will present samples of the raw statistics using a range of methods. The question of which statistic is most useful depends on your point of view. For example, doctors working in public health, responsible for planning healthcare provision for a local population, will not be very interested in the rates of a given cancer in another country. Conversely, researchers looking at the effect of diet on risk of cancer may well want to focus on differences in disease rates between societies, as they may shed light on which lifestyle factors are important in the development of a given cancer. Fundraisers for cancer research will tend to focus on diseases affecting large numbers in the target donating population – breast cancer is the best example of this in Europe and North America, but more recently fundraising for prostate cancer has tapped into the same vein of public opinion.

The raw figures

As already mentioned, around 13%, or 1 in 7, of all deaths worldwide are due to cancer. This rises to around 1 in 3–4 in the developed world, where risk of premature death from infections, malnutrition, or violence is comparatively much lower. Figure 1 shows the numbers diagnosed with, and Figures 2 and 3 those dying from, cancer in different parts of the world. It is clear that there are large variations by region, with cancers common in one part of the world not featuring in the list of common cancers in another. There are too many differences to cover every one in detail. I will therefore highlight a few to illustrate why and how these differences arise.

Lung cancer

Worldwide, lung cancer is the largest cause of cancer death, with 17% of all cancer deaths, amounting to 1.2 million people, due to this type. It is a highly lethal disease, with fewer than 1 in 10 diagnosed surviving 5 years in most countries. Even in the United States, which has the best treatment results, fewer than 1 in 5 survive long term. Furthermore, the worldwide death rate is rising rapidly, having doubled between 1975 and 2002. Figure 1 shows the rates of diagnosis for different cancers around the world and clearly shows that lung cancer is among the major killers in all parts of the globe. There is a well-known, strong link between smoking and lung cancer. Differences in the rates of lung cancer not surprisingly therefore vary with rates of smoking. Mostly, lung cancer is diagnosed relatively late in life, reflecting consumption of large numbers of cigarettes over half a century in most cases (younger people who have had less exposure obviously can suffer from the disease, but these cases are relatively less common). It therefore follows that the rates of lung cancer and the trend in the rates (rising or falling) reflect smoking habits over the previous half century. If we know the trends in rates of smoking, we can predict the future trends in lung cancer rates for a population.

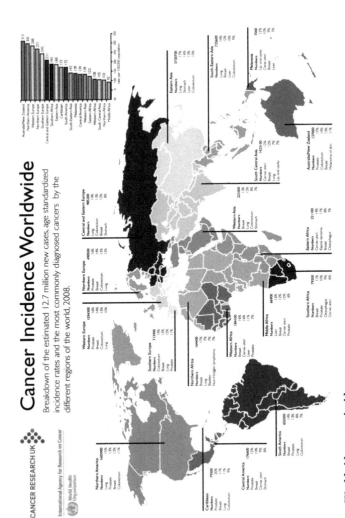

Cancer Incidence Worldwide

Breakdown of the estimated 12.7 million new cases, age standardized incidence rates and the most commonly diagnosed cancers by the different regions of the world, 2008.

CANCER RESEARCH UK

International Agency for Research on Cancer
World Health Organization

Northern America
1460900
Numbers
Prostate 15%
Breast 14%
Lung 13%
Colorectum 11%

Caribbean
79000
Numbers
Prostate 16%
Breast 13%
Lung 11%
Colorectum 9%

Central America
176600
Numbers
Breast 13%
Prostate 12%
Cervix uteri 9%
Stomach 8%

South America
650300
Numbers
Breast 14%
Prostate 13%
Cervix uteri 9%
Colorectum 7%

Western Europe
1054300
Numbers
Prostate 16%
Breast 14%
Colorectum 13%
Lung 10%

Northern Europe
495500
Numbers
Prostate 16%
Breast 14%
Colorectum 13%
Lung 12%

Southern Europe
719900
Numbers
Colorectum 13%
Breast 12%
Lung 12%
Prostate 11%

Central and Eastern Europe
980300
Numbers
Lung 14%
Colorectum 13%
Breast 12%
Stomach 8%

Northern Africa
164400
Numbers
Breast 17%
Bladder 7%
Liver 7%
Non-Hodgkin lymphoma 7%

Western Africa
184100
Numbers
Breast 16%
Cervix uteri 16%
Liver 10%
Prostate 7%

Middle Africa
66100
Numbers
Cervix uteri 16%
Breast 12%
Prostate 8%

Southern Africa
79000
Numbers
Breast 11%
Prostate 11%
Oesophagus 10%
Cervix uteri 8%

Eastern Africa
221100
Numbers
Cervix uteri 21%
Kaposi sarcoma 11%
Breast 8%
Oesophagus 7%

Western Asia
223300
Numbers
Breast 18%
Lung 8%
Colorectum 8%
Stomach 7%

Eastern Asia
3720700
Numbers
Lung 17%
Stomach 14%
Liver 12%
Colorectum 10%

South-Eastern Asia
725600
Numbers
Lung 14%
Breast 13%
Liver 10%
Colorectum 9%

South Central Asia
1423100
Numbers
Cervix uteri 13%
Breast 13%
Lung 8%
Lip, oral cavity 7%

Australia/New Zealand
127000
Numbers
Prostate 17%
Colorectum 14%
Breast 14%
Melanoma of skin 11%

Melanesia
7900
Numbers
Lip, oral cavity 23%
Breast 13%
Liver 9%
Lung 7%

1. Worldwide cancer incidence

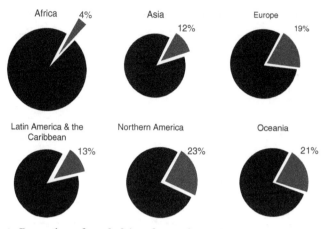

2. Proportions of people dying of cancer by continent

In Western Europe and North America, rates of smoking in men are declining and with them rates of lung cancer (and other smoking-related diseases). In contrast, in large tracts of the developing world, rates of smoking are increasing rapidly as countries industrialize. The effect this is likely to have on cancer rates is illustrated by trends in Japan, where the rate of lung cancer between 1960 and 1980 more than doubled as the effects of Japan's industrialization took their toll. Similar changes are now being observed in countries like China. There are various reasons for this: the habit still has an aura of 'coolness' in these countries very different from the increasing pariah status of smokers in the West. There are generally lower levels of awareness of the health issues attached to smoking, and the restrictions on tobacco promotion increasingly seen in Europe and North America are not present. Indeed, officials in one recession-hit Chinese province recently decreed that all adults had to smoke the local cigarettes in order to boost both the local growers and tax revenues. Looking forwards, therefore, we can see that just as lung cancer declines as

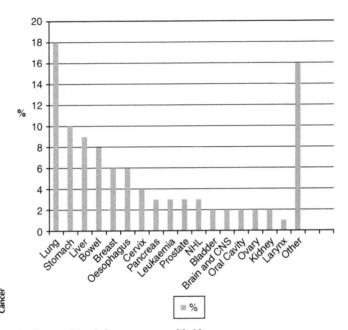

3. Causes of death from cancer worldwide

a problem in the 'developed' world, the newly industrializing economies will face an increasing burden of smoking-related cancers (and other problems such as heart disease) unless there is rapid adoption of the sorts of smoking-prevention strategies now the norm in Western Europe and North America. At present, this seems unlikely, and thus the industrializing world is likely to acquire one of the less desirable trappings of the developed world.

Breast cancer

In terms of new cases, breast cancer is the commonest cancer in women, accounting for 21% of female cancer cases and 14% of

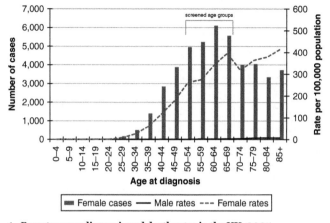

4. Breast cancer diagnosis and death rates in the UK, 2005

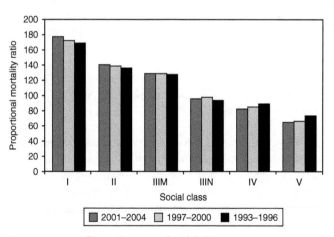

5. Breast cancer diagnosis rates and social class

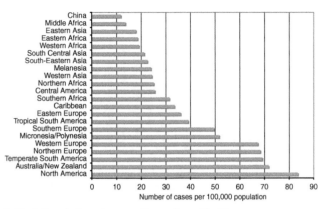

6. Variations in breast cancer diagnosis worldwide

female cancer deaths worldwide. The overall survival rate is, however, much better than for lung cancer, with three-quarters of sufferers in Europe and North America surviving 5 years. Even in less developed countries, over half of breast cancer patients will reach this milestone.

A study of the patterns of occurrence of breast cancer also helps to illustrate some of the ways cancer statistics can shed light on the behaviour of the disease.

The risk of getting breast cancer (as for most cancers) increases steadily with age, illustrated in Figure 4 with data from the UK. Very similar distributions will be found in all developed countries. If we look at the left-hand axis in the figure – the actual numbers for each age – the peak numbers occur in the 50–70 age range – although their risk is higher, there are fewer women in the 70+ age groups due to deaths from other causes. As can also be seen, few women aged under 40 are diagnosed with the disease, although fundraisers often use women from this age group in their promotional materials. The second figure, Figure 5, looks at the distribution of cases from another angle, that of social class. This demonstrates that wealthier, better-educated women are at significantly higher risk than the less well off. Middle-aged educated women are often formidable campaigners, having both the time and education to lobby effectively. As we shall see later in the book, neither cancer research nor treatment access are arranged purely on the basis of need but are often substantially influenced by lobby-group pressure on behalf of particular groups.

The figures on worldwide risk of breast cancer again show some striking trends. Looking at Figure 5, there is a clear suggestion that breast cancer is in some way associated with affluence – richer countries have higher rates than poorer ones. For the smoking/cancer link, there is a pretty clear relationship between consumption and risk. It is harder to see why higher average income should increase the risk of an illness – this is the reverse of most public health trends. So why should this be? One factor is the age structure of the population. As seen in Figure 4, risk of cancer increases with age. Hence a woman in a poor country with a low life expectancy may simply not live long enough to get breast cancer, having already died of another disease earlier in life. This does not account for the large range of risk seen, however. There are various theories about the observed underlying difference, and the most likely explanation relates to the effect of hormones on the breast tissue. For example, there are clear effects on cancer risk relating to age of first pregnancy and numbers of pregnancies. Late onset of puberty, early first pregnancy, and more frequent pregnancies are factors that appear to protect against breast cancer. In the West, puberty occurs earlier than in the past due to better nutrition and higher-protein diets, whereas pregnancy occurs later due to effective contraception, the increasing independence of women, and better education. In poorer countries, puberty occurs later and women have less control over their fertility. Whilst this situation of course brings all sorts of potential problems, it does appear to protect against breast cancer. Breast-feeding, which affects hormone levels post-delivery, also appears to protect against breast cancer, and being more prevalent among the better educated in the West may be predicted to skew the trend the other way. Fertility rates tend to drop and age at first pregnancy tends to rise as both national and personal income increases, so it may be expected that, as with lung cancer, increasing development will result in an increase in cases of breast cancer worldwide.

Clearly, the breast is an organ that changes throughout life in response to changes in hormone levels (arising from puberty, pregnancy, breast-feeding, menopause, or drug therapies such as oral contraception and hormone replacement therapy). It follows from the above observations that medical treatments that affect hormone levels may alter the risk of developing breast cancer. Hormone replacement therapy (HRT) is widely used for menopausal symptoms. It was hoped that, in addition to helping ameliorate symptoms such as hot flushes and loss of libido, HRT would prevent diseases that tend to occur with increasing frequency after the menopause such as heart disease and bone loss (osteoporosis) with consequent risk of fracture. While HRT is indeed effective in some of these aims, it also appears to increase risk of breast cancer with prolonged use. A similar effect is seen with the oral contraceptive pill, which again works by altering the normal hormone environment. These, then, are confusing effects: some hormone changes (those associated with pregnancy and breast-feeding) protect against breast cancer, while other changes (oral contraception and HRT) increase risk. Against this background, much laboratory research is focused on the role that hormones play in the causation of breast cancer and on the development of drugs that interfere with hormone pathways and thereby treat breast cancer. One of these drugs, tamoxifen, which acts mainly by blocking the effects of the hormone oestrogen, can be regarded as one of the most effective drugs of all time, having saved the lives of probably millions of women and helped prolong life for many more in the 25 or so years since it came into clinical use (see Chapter 3).

Finally, there is a perception, promoted to a degree by groups campaigning for better treatment and research, that breast cancer is a disease of young women. In general, as we have already seen, this is inaccurate. However, studies of patterns of risk of breast cancer revealed that some families appear to be at very high risk of breast cancer, with mothers, sisters, aunts all affected at an early age, often with disease in both breasts or associated with cancer of the ovaries, or of the prostate in the male relatives. These families were obvious candidates for in-depth study and, given the very obvious risks to the families involved, sufferers were often very receptive to participation in research. Studies of the patterns of inheritance in such cases suggested that the risk of breast cancer was passed on from mother to child with a 50:50 risk, and suggested at least two common inherited forms of the disease plus a number of less common versions. This is an area of research covered in more detail in Chapter 2.

Liver cancer

Liver cancer is one of the commonest cancers worldwide but with a very different pattern of distribution to lung and breast cancer. It is of particular interest as a freely available vaccination (against hepatitis B) can effectively prevent development of the cancer. Overall, it is the sixth most common cancer in terms of new cases, but the third most common cause of cancer death, reflecting the highly aggressive nature of the disease. There are a number of key features to the pattern of cases of liver cancer that merit more detailed examination. It is between 5 and 7 times more common in parts of China and Africa than in Europe and North America. The disease is almost always lethal, partly because it occurs in parts of the world with less developed healthcare, but mostly because it arises as a result of serious damage to the liver by the hepatitis B virus.

Liver cancer is linked to chronic liver damage, and in Europe and North America this is generally caused by alcohol abuse. In the parts of the world where the cancer is more common, the more important factor is infection with the hepatitis B virus (HBV), first described in 1965 by Dr Baruch Blumberg, who received the Nobel Prize for his work. Epidemiological studies established the link between hepatitis and liver cancer some years ago. Subsequent work showed that the molecular biology of the virus was consistent with it having a direct causative role rather than this being a chance association. With the linkage between virus and cancer established, the possibility of a vaccine against a common cancer became a reality. Pleasingly for all concerned, HBV vaccination has been a great success, with benefits appearing in the highest-risk populations very rapidly.

Cancers of the gut

Gut cancers commonly occur either in the top end (stomach and oesophagus) or the bottom end (colon and rectum), with cancers of the middle bit (the small bowel) being comparatively rare. There are some interesting trends in the patterns of gut cancers which I will run through, starting at the top with stomach cancer.

Overall, almost a million people are diagnosed with stomach cancer each year with around two-thirds of those afflicted dying from the disease – at least 650,000. Stomach cancer has been steadily falling in incidence in the West over the last 50 years, as illustrated in Figure 7, moving from being a relatively common cancer to now being quite rare. In other parts of the world, incidence has also begun to fall but more recently. Various reasons have been proposed for this, ranging from the rise of cheap refrigerators to medical treatments for stomach ulceration, but at present the reasons for the changes are not fully understood.

Cancers of the large bowel also show large variations between populations. Broadly speaking, bowel cancer is common in Europe and North America, less common in the Far East and uncommon in Africa. It is thus predominantly a disease of the developed world. Altogether, around a million people are diagnosed with the disease each year, and around half of these

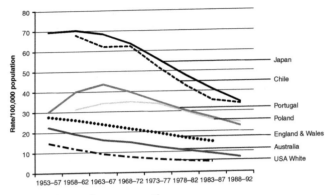

7. **Rates of stomach cancer over time**

patients will die from the disease. Death rates are now declining in North America and Europe due to improved awareness, early diagnosis, and better treatment. Studies of migrants suggest that the differences are environmental rather than racial – migrants from low-risk to high-risk countries rapidly take on the risk pattern of their new homeland. In addition, countries with an increasingly Westernized diet such as Japan are seeing a rise in the incidence of the disease. The prime candidate for this effect is therefore diet – differences in the environment of the lining of the lower bowel clearly arise from differences in what goes in at the top end! There thus appears to be some sort of reciprocal effect – changes in diet over the last 50 years have made stomach cancer increasingly rare but have led to an increased risk of cancer at the other end of the bowel. Studying these sorts of changes provides important clues to the origins of cancers and also can point the way to prevention strategies.

Prostate cancer

Prostate cancer is an interesting disease. In Europe and North America, it is the most frequently diagnosed cancer in men and one of the leading causes of cancer death in men. In 2007, worldwide there were 670,000 men diagnosed with the disease. Deaths are more difficult to ascertain as many men diagnosed with early prostate cancer die with rather than of the disease. Like breast cancer, there are major differences in rates between different countries. Some of these differences appear to be driven by differences in rates of use of a blood test for prostate-specific antigen (PSA) which will detect early cancers and can be used as a screening test.

Prostate-specific antigen is made by the prostate and is a protein whose normal function is to liquefy the fluid produced during ejaculation (an aside – rodents do not make PSA and produce a solid semen plug during intercourse, yet mice are widely used in prostate cancer research). PSA is found in small quantities in the blood in men without cancer. In the presence of a prostate cancer (but also in other diseases affecting the prostate), larger amounts are liberated into the bloodstream, enabling the measurement of PSA to be used as both an early diagnostic and monitoring test for prostate cancer. Since the early 1990s, the test has been increasingly widely available and used both for screening for undiagnosed cancer and as a tool for monitoring the response of the cancer to treatment. In the USA, the test has been widely available from a range of sources and is actively promoted to the public by the makers of test kits – knowledge of your PSA level has become something men need to be aware of in the same way that cholesterol used to be. In the UK, until recently, government policy discouraged 'opportunistic' PSA testing, and there was no systematic screening programme on the grounds that there was no evidence that early diagnosis of prostate cancer reduced death rates from the disease. Recent data from screening trials suggest that PSA testing may reduce deaths from prostate cancer, but that around 40 men need to be treated for PSA-test-detected cancer in order to save 1 life. Whether this level of benefit will result in screening programmes being set up remains to be seen. It should be noted that this is similar to the level of benefit from breast cancer screening. Although widely applied, the benefits of screening are therefore not nearly as clear cut as may be imagined from the very widespread application of breast cancer screening across the Western world. For the time being, PSA testing is variable across the world and largely consumer driven.

If we start by looking at diagnosis and death rates from prostate cancer, some very obvious differences are seen (Figure 8). Men living in Europe and North America have a strikingly higher death rate than men living in Indo-China, where the disease is relatively rare, as it is also in most of Africa. Within Europe and North America, there are further interesting variations, with increasing risk of death with increasing distance from the Equator, an effect best seen in the white populations of the United States and Australia where the ethnicity of the white population is fairly uniform. If we look at ethnic effects, there are also striking variations, with men of African origin having roughly double the risk of prostate cancer death than white men. In contrast, men of Indo-Chinese descent retain the lower risk of their regions of origin, similar to the effect seen with women and breast cancer.

How can we explain this? The best evidence suggests that the differences between the white and Asian populations are driven by differences in diet plus a difference in racial sensitivity to whatever causes prostate cancer (which is largely unknown). The variation with latitude is much harder to explain by diet and clearly is not explained by race, as it can be observed in Europe, North America, and Australia. The best explanation seems to be exposure to sunlight, with sun exposure being protective. This is a very surprising conclusion, given the widespread public health campaigns aimed at reducing people's exposure to the sun. How may sun exposure affect the risk of cancer in an internal organ about as protected from the sun as it is possible to be? The answer appears to be vitamin D. Lack of vitamin D leads to rickets and conjures up images of Victorian workhouses and deformed children, but the 21st-century version of the disease may be an increased risk of cancer, as summarized in the box.

Vitamin D, sunlight, and cancer

Vitamin D is closely involved in the growth and development of a whole range of tissues including glandular structures like the prostate and breast. Vitamin D metabolism is complex, but a key step occurs in the skin and requires sunlight. Lack of exposure to sunlight over prolonged periods may thus lead to a shortage of 'active' vitamin D – not enough to cause rickets, but enough to shade the odds of getting prostate cancer. This may also explain why men of African origin, who often have the darkest skins, may be at the highest risk of prostate cancer if living in temperate latitudes. If this hypothesis were true, it could be predicted that white people with the highest sun exposure in a population would have a lower risk of prostate cancer. A good index of sun exposure is skin cancer, and studies have been carried out of prostate cancer risk in those with skin cancer. As predicted, the risk of prostate cancer is reduced in those with the highest levels of sun exposure as evidenced by solar skin damage and skin cancer. What is more, with sun exposure, reduction in an individual's risk of getting prostate cancer is substantial – one study estimates this may be as much as 40%. Even in those developing prostate cancer, sun exposure appears to delay diagnosis significantly – around 5 years, from an average age of 67 years for the least sun-exposed to 72 for the most sun-exposed. The central message thus appears to be very consistent – one of the biggest killers of the male population could be prevented by more sunbathing – yet public health policy advises against it!

If this effect is present with prostate cancer, clearly mediated by circulating factors generated in the skin, could it be seen with other cancers as well? The answer appears to be 'yes', and the effect size seems to be similar for pretty much all cancers of internal organs. The only cancers that are increased by sun exposure are those of the skin (specifically melanoma), which

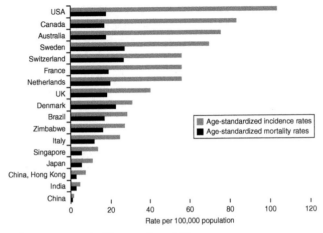

8. Prostate cancer incidence and mortality

actually kill relatively few people. The study of prostate cancer death rates thus sheds all sorts of interesting light on the causation of common cancers, and has thrown up a very surprising connection that fundamentally challenges current standard public health advice. In the opinion of the author, the accepted wisdom on sun exposure is overdue for radical revision.

There is a second striking set of differences in the diagnosis and death rates. If we compare, say, the UK and the USA, we see very similar death rates but very different diagnosis rates per 100,000 population, with more than twice as many cases diagnosed per death from prostate cancer in the USA as in the UK. Looked at another way, a far lower percentage of men with prostate cancer die from the disease in the USA than in the UK.

There are a number of possible explanations – prostate cancer may truly be more common in the USA, and the US healthcare system twice as good at treating it as the UK system. Whilst it is true that the UK healthcare system delivers slightly inferior outcomes compared to the US system, these differences for most cancers are of the order of a few percentage points and are unlikely to explain the apparent difference in cure rates. Furthermore, if we look at rates of detection for other common cancers, the UK and USA have generally similar numbers per 100,000 population, suggesting that other factors are operating. The explanation lies in the PSA blood test.

Differences in public policy and availability of PSA tests have resulted in far fewer men being tested in the UK than the USA, with a consequently lower rate of diagnosis of the disease. However, most men diagnosed in the USA, where there are high rates of PSA blood testing, have clinically trivial disease. This may never have troubled them had they not been diagnosed with it, suggesting the large difference in incidence is largely driven by higher rates of diagnosis of low-grade, relatively non-lethal disease in the USA compared to the UK. Both sides of the Atlantic, a smaller number of men are diagnosed and eventually die from more aggressive forms of the disease. Since the late 1990s, death rates have been falling, but whether this is down to screening directly or to other factors is hotly debated.

Politics of cancer care

There are clearly many angles to the politics of cancer care, and these are linked closely to the economics of the disease. For the purposes of this chapter, I will focus on the differences in cases diagnosed and death rates and how they drive the politics of the disease, using breast and prostate cancer to illustrate gender differences and breast and lung cancer to illustrate social class effects.

In many ways, prostate cancer is the male counterpart of breast cancer. The similarities extend to a number of levels: both organs have a role in sexuality and reproduction; both change during life in response to hormone levels; both cancers can be treated by changes in the hormone environment; and treatments for the cancers arising in the respective organs cause profound changes in sexual function. Politically, the powerful sexual and emotional imagery of the breast has been used to great effect to channel research and treatment funds into breast cancer for many decades. This has resulted in steady and progressive improvement in outcomes for women with breast cancer, reflected both in improved survival and reduced damage from successful treatment. For example, women are increasingly offered less mutilating surgery or breast reconstructions rather than radical mastectomy. On the drug funding issue, women have again been very effective at campaigning for new treatments – witness the rapid uptake of trastuzumab (better known as Herceptin) across the European and North American healthcare systems.

Until recently, despite the biological parallels, there was no analogous movement to support men with prostate cancer or campaigning to improve treatments and outcomes. As recently as 1995, for example, spending on prostate cancer research in the UK was only one-tenth that on breast cancer. In the last 10 years, this has changed, partly driven by the PSA test. This shifted the spectrum of prostate cancer substantially to the 'left', with a decrease in late cases and increase in early cases for which the treatment options are more varied and the possibility exists for cure or prolonged survival with the disease. This historical lack of public health and research interest is particularly surprising given the general concentration of political and economic power in the hands of men of middle age and above – those most at risk of the disease and with very little risk of breast cancer (though men can get it). The difference appears to be rooted in the differing psychologies of men and women – it's fine for women to talk about breast cancer, and women are not seen as diminished but often rather strengthened by it – witness Kylie Minogue's recent world tour. On the other hand, it has previously been very difficult for men to talk about the disease, particularly when treatments carry 'unmacho' risks such as impotence and incontinence, quite apart from the fundamentally embarrassing route needed for diagnosis (via the rectum). Coupled with most men's general 'ostrich' approach to all matters related to health, the result has been a price paid by men living shorter, less healthy lives than women.

More recently, however, there has been a shift in public and economic policies, with more money spent on treatment for men and research into the disease. This has been driven no doubt in part by the pharmaceutical industry's belated realization that there is a lot of money to be made from one of the biggest male cancer killers in the West. There has also been a change in that major public figures such as Colin Powell, Roger Moore, and Rudolph Giuliani have been prepared to talk about their treatment for the disease.

Finally, the issue of smoking and public policy is worth mentioning in the context of the politics of cancer care, as this has varied widely across the world and over the decades. Not too long ago, tobacco companies actually ran adverts with the strap-line that a particular cigarette was the preferred brand for doctors. The linkage of smoking to increased risk of various cancers has been one of the triumphs of epidemiological research, and has resulted in massive reductions in the rates of smoking and diseases linked to it in the developed world. A range of measures has driven this, from legal (smoking bans) through educational (advertising and sponsorship bans, health warnings) through to fiscal (tax the stuff, which has the additional benefit of paying for the healthcare needed to pick up the consequences for smokers). In the developing world, things are different, however: smoking is still seen as 'cool', underpinned by advertising and marketing to young people, rather than the pariah activity banished to chilly doorways it has increasingly become in Europe and North America. Furthermore, the money brought in to developing countries by the big multinational tobacco companies carries with it much political clout, and this can used to tone down the public health assault on the habit that has occurred in the West. Coupled with the young age structures of developing countries, an epidemic of developing world smoking-related cancers – lung, bladder, throat, mouth – can be anticipated in the coming years. In countries like China which are rapidly modernizing and improving living standards and life expectancy, this can be expected to result in particularly large increases in these cancers.

Chapter 2
How does cancer develop?

In order to understand how cancer develops, it is necessary to include a little background on basic cell biology. The cell is the basic building block that makes up all living things. The human body, in common with all animals from the smallest such as yeast to the largest blue whale, is composed of cells. Some animals – yeast, for example – are made of single cells; others, ourselves included, are made of many different sorts of cells – blood, bone, brain, kidney, and so on. All cells in an organism have their own carefully controlled life cycle. Cancer occurs when the control of this cycle goes wrong, leading to unregulated growth of a group of cells which can spread and damage other structures in the body. This chapter will focus on how cancer develops and also on some of the underlying biology needed to understand this. I will also illustrate how an understanding of the causes can be used to define treatment strategies.

The key component of the cell for understanding cancer is the nucleus, which holds the DNA that contains the genetic code. Figure 9 shows a diagram of a DNA molecule. Cancer is caused fundamentally by damage to the DNA leading to abnormal, unregulated growth of cells. Remarkably, although different cells may differ markedly in their appearance and function (for example, nerve cells, muscle cells, and blood cells), all the cells in a given organism share the same DNA code. DNA is clustered into long strands called chromosomes. There are 23 pairs in each human cell. Within each chromosome, the DNA is arranged in genes, each one coding for a single protein. We can think about genes and chromosomes as being like a library of books, with each of the 23 chromosomes an individual volume and each of the 21,000 genes a page of instructions in that volume. It is easy to see conceptually how damage to a page of instructions can lead to alterations in the properties of a cell. This chapter will run through how these different structures work and interact, and how they can go wrong to lead to the development of a cancer.

Everyone starts life as a single fertilized egg that develops first into a ball of identical cells and then, progressively, grows, organizes, and develops into a complete complex individual. The process by which cells develop from this initial group into highly specialized subtypes is one of the most incredibly complex processes in nature and yet is happening constantly all around us and within us. This clearly requires an intricate network of checks and balances. It requires that cells communicate with their neighbours to ensure that the right development path is followed at the right time. It requires that cells no longer required are deleted and eliminated with the minimum of disruption (a process called apoptosis, from the Greek word meaning 'a falling off of petals'). As organs develop, they must grow their own blood supplies and maintain them in response to damage. It requires that organ systems communicate with each other, for example nerves connecting with the muscles they control. Endocrine (hormone) glands are coordinated to produce their products in cycles (for example, the ovaries) or in response to stress (the adrenal glands). This is achieved by genes being switched on and off in a coordinated fashion as individual organ systems grow and develop. Once the growth process is complete and the animal is formed, tissues must be maintained, damage repaired, and general housekeeping kept ticking over – nutrients supplied and processed, waste products eliminated, and so on. The more one thinks about the

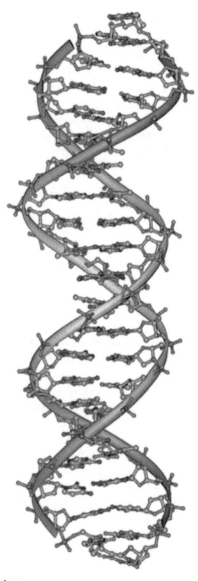

9. DNA structure

mind-blowing complexity of all these tasks, the remarkable thing is that the processes run so reliably for so many years in most people, and that cancer – essentially, unregulated cell division – does not occur more frequently than it does.

DNA structure and function

As already mentioned, the genetic code is stored in human cells in 23 pairs of chromosomes. Each chromosome comprises a very long molecule of DNA containing the genes, which are interspersed with spacer sequences. Each gene is flanked by regions of DNA that control when a particular gene is switched on or off. For example, the gene coding for the protein myosin, a key component of muscle cells, will be switched on where needed – in muscle – but off in other tissues where it is not required, such as nerve cells. The network of on and off switches is clearly critical to regulation of the behaviour of cells, and study of these controls is a major feature of cancer research – if the controls do not work, cells can grow in an unregulated fashion, as occurs in cancers.

To understand how cells carry out all these functions, it is necessary to understand a bit more about the structure of DNA and how the code embedded in the DNA molecule is translated into the end product that is the functioning organism. DNA is an abbreviation for deoxyribose nucleic acid. It had been known for some time before the famous discovery of its double helical structure by Crick and Watson in 1953 that DNA contained the genetic code. The DNA molecule (illustrated in Figure 9) is a long spine of two alternating building blocks – a sugar (called deoxyribose) and a phosphate group linked to four molecules named adenine, guanine, cytosine, and thymine (abbreviated to A, G, C, T) and referred to as bases. These bases are arranged along the spine of the DNA molecule and form two complementary pairs, A with T and C with G, that can bond to each other. The double helical nature of DNA results from one strand (the positive or sense strand) being matched by a complementary antisense strand with an A paired with every T, C with every G, and so on. The A–T and C–G bonds thus provide the 'glue' that maintains the double helical structure of the DNA strands. The complementary nature of the bond process means that if the two strands are pulled apart and each used as a template for two new strands, the result is two identical copies of the first DNA molecule.

This inherent property of DNA, whereby it can make identical copies of itself, is one of the fundamental properties of all life on Earth. The structure of DNA is very tightly conserved across the whole spectrum from the simplest to the most complex. The fidelity of the duplication process is also extremely high. The error rate is so low that it takes many generations to accumulate significant differences – the rate of genetic 'drift' – and is one of the bases for evolutionary biology. Coming back to the genetic books in the library: each time a cell divides, a complete set of the 23 pairs of volumes with their 21,000 genes ('pages' of information) must be 'typed' by the cell. From time to time, a comma, letter, or full stop will be mistyped. Mostly, as in a book, this will not alter the meaning, but sometimes, changes will be critical, with consequent alteration to how the daughter cell carrying the change (called a mutation) functions. Parenthetically, the number of small random differences can be tracked across the evolutionary tree to allow estimates of when a given pair of species diverged from each other.

Genes and control of gene expression

The fundamental unit that the DNA is organized around is the gene. A gene contains the code for a single protein. Proteins can have many functions ranging from structural, for example a protein called tubulin which makes the cell's internal 'skeleton', to functional, such as forming the parts of muscles that contract. This flow of information, whereby information in DNA is transcribed into a message (in RNA) and then into a single protein, is one of the central concepts of biology.

Proteins are the key building blocks of cells, responsible for all the key activities. Other components of cells, such as fats and sugars, are manufactured as a result of actions of proteins. Proteins clearly have to have a range of functions, therefore. These include: signalling both within and between cells; structure (a sort of microscopic scaffolding); and, very importantly, proteins called enzymes, which act on other biological molecules to bring about the formation of new molecules. This process can be destructive – for example, the enzymes in digestive secretions (and washing powders!) which break down food; or constructive – the enzymes involved in the manufacture of new molecules for the cell.

The production of a protein from a gene involves the transcription of the gene into a messenger ribose nucleic acid (mRNA) molecule within the nucleus of the cell. The RNA molecule has a structure like DNA but differs in key respects. Firstly, the deoxyribose sugar (the D in DNA) in the backbone is replaced by ribose (the R in RNA). Secondly, the molecule is single-stranded. And thirdly, the thymine (T) base is substituted by uracil (U), though the pairing remains the same.

In order to make RNA, the DNA double helix is temporarily 'unzipped' into two single strands. A complementary RNA molecule then assembles and is transported out of the nucleus into the cytoplasm and the DNA then zips itself back up again. This process, another key part of biology, is called transcription and is illustrated in Figure 10.

Once in the cytoplasm, this messenger RNA must be converted into protein, the second key part of the translation of the code embedded in the DNA into functional proteins. A second sort of RNA – called transfer RNA – provides the link between the messenger RNA and the building blocks of protein. Key to this translation process is the triplet code embedded in the DNA. Proteins, like DNA, are made up of chains of simpler molecules. The protein building blocks, called amino acids, can be linked

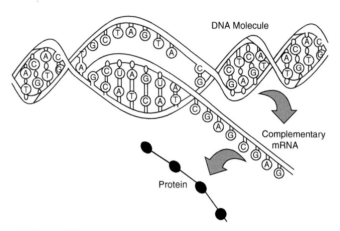

10. Transcription

together to form effectively endless chains. The basic amino acid molecule has three key features – termed a carboxy terminus and an amino (hence the name) terminus, plus a variable side branch which gives each amino acid its distinct properties (illustrated as R in Figure 11).

Whilst in theory an infinite number of types of amino acids are possible, only 20 are found in living organisms. The DNA code is arranged in triplets called codons. There are 64 possible three-letter codes using A, T/U, C, and G. Each triplet has a specific meaning and can either refer to an amino acid or, in effect, form a punctuation mark. For example, within this coding system, AUG means 'start here' (termed a 'start codon'); UAG, UGA, and UAA mean 'stop here'; while the remainder are linked to specific amino acids – for example, cysteine is UGU or UGC. As there are 64 possible combinations in the triple code but only 20 amino acids, it follows that some amino acids have more than one triplet code. It can easily be seen, therefore, that a mutation which changes a single base can fundamentally alter the resultant protein. For example, a

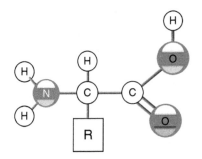

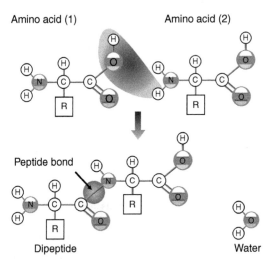

Amino acid (1)   Amino acid (2)

Peptide bond

Dipeptide   Water

11. Amino acids and protein structure

change from UGC (cysteine) to UGA (the stop signal) will shorten the resultant protein, with a possible major change in function.

As already mentioned, the core code of the gene is flanked by complex regulatory machinery (see Figure 12) to ensure genes are switched on and off at the correct times. It is this regulation of gene function that is often faulty in the cancer cell.

Regulation of gene expression requires the interaction of a complex series of events. To understand this, a little more detail on gene structure is required (see Figure 12).

On both sides of the coding portion of a gene are the control regions. As with a mutation in the coding region described already, it can easily be understood how changes to the regulation of the gene or the processing of the messenger RNA can result in over- or under-production of a protein or the generation of an abnormal protein with undesirable properties. These control regions are themselves regulated by other genes, called transcription factors, which turn gene expression up or down like a volume control. The transcription factors are the key regulators of the whole process, and it is therefore unsurprising that many of the genes involved in cancer turn out to be from this family of proteins.

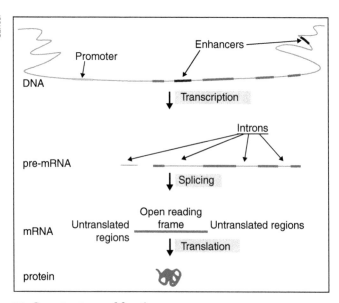

12. **Gene structure and function**

The hallmarks of cancer

Having covered the basics of the machinery, we can now turn to the ways in which the processes go wrong to produce a cancer. In 2000, two leading cell biologists, Douglas Hanahan and Robert Weinberg, published a seminal paper entitled 'The Hallmarks of Cancer' summarizing the changes that are both necessary and sufficient to produce a cancer. A cancer cell differs from normal cells in that it divides in an unregulated fashion. In addition, cancer cells have the ability to spread to and invade other parts of the body. Hanahan and Weinberg summarized the processes that must occur in the cell in order for it to be transformed from a normal, law-abiding member of cellular society into a dangerous outlaw. These changes, illustrated in Figure 13, are characterized as:

- self-sufficiency in positive growth signals;
- lack of response to inhibitory signals;
- failure to undergo 'programmed cell death' to eliminate faulty cells;
- evasion of destruction by the immune system;
- the ability to grow in and destructively invade other tissues;
- ability to sustain growth by generating new blood vessels.

The first two of these are reasonably self-explanatory and lead to unregulated growth. The third is less obvious and is linked to the development process. If all cells simply grew and divided, it would not be possible, for example, to form hollow tubular structures such as the gut or blood vessels. To do this, certain cells must be deleted from the growing organism as the needs of the growing structure dictate. This process, already mentioned, is called apoptosis, and is a key cellular function. Apoptosis is also a method that the organism uses to get rid of faulty or malfunctioning cells such as those nearing the end of their lifespan that need replacing. Cancer cells are by definition abnormal and thus should be self-deleting. Failure to undergo apoptosis is thus key to the transformation from an abnormal cell into one with limitless replicative potential. A further feature of apoptosis is that cells damaged by chemotherapy or radiotherapy

13. The hallmarks of cancer

are frequently not killed outright, but merely 'mortally wounded'. The subsequent death of the cell is often by apoptosis, illustrating that the evasion mechanism is not completely shut down, even in the cancer cell. Increasing resistance to apoptosis is, however, one way in which the cancer cell evades destruction by chemotherapy or radiotherapy (see Chapter 3). Understanding apoptosis is unsurprisingly therefore one of the major areas of cancer research.

Further distinguishing features of cancers are their ability to grow and to invade other tissues in the body while avoiding destruction themselves by the immune system. The immune system can be regarded as a sort of cellular police force that identifies intruders such as bacteria and eliminates them. As cancer cells are abnormal, the immune system should be able to identify and destroy them. Evasion of this process is therefore essential to the cancer. As already indicated, the growth and development of cells, tissues, and organs is very finely regulated to ensure the correct sort of cell grows in the correct place and time in the organism. One key aspect of cancer growth is the acquisition of the ability to grow in the wrong place, and this is a feature that distinguishes a malignant tumour from a benign one, which can grow but not spread or invade. It should be noted that benign tumours can still present severe consequences, for example an acoustic neuroma is a benign tumour of the auditory nerve that transmits signals from the inner ear to the brain. The tumour will progressively enlarge, causing deafness and balance problems, without ever spreading elsewhere.

The final hallmark of cancer is the ability to grow a new blood supply. Any collection of cells larger than around one-tenth of a millimetre across needs a blood supply. As the new tumour grows, it must therefore acquire the ability to stimulate blood vessel growth. The blood vessel growth of tumours is often haphazard and turns out to use genes not involved in the maintenance of normal blood vessels. The process is known as tumour angiogenesis, and because it differs from normal angiogenesis, it has become an important target for cancer drug development. If it is possible to knock out the blood supply of the cancer, further growth is prevented. One of the most successful of the new generation of targeted molecular therapies, bevacizumab (Avastin), works by targeting this process.

Carcinogenesis – how cancers start

As already indicated, cancer results when the changes required for the hallmarks of cancer have occurred. To understand how cancer develops, we now need to turn to how external factors bring about cancer – a process known as carcinogenesis. Fundamentally, cancer results from damage to DNA, leading to the changes described above and illustrated in Figure 13. All agents that damage DNA therefore are potential carcinogens – agents that cause cancer. The reverse is not true, however; not all agents that help cause cancer themselves directly damage DNA, though this always lies at the end of the process. Examples of cancer-causing substances that do not directly damage DNA include alcohol and the sex hormones involved in causing breast and prostate cancer. There are many sorts of carcinogens and many are well known – cigarette smoke and ionizing radiation, for example. Taking cigarette smoking, we know that typically it is necessary to smoke many cigarettes for many years for cancer to develop. This suggests that the process of carcinogenesis is slow and potentially has more than one step. From the discussion above, it would be predicted that mutations would be necessary in different sets of genes to cause the hallmark changes described by Hanahan and Weinberg. Such a chain of events was also postulated in the early 1990s and is now often referred to as the 'Vogelstein cascade', with each step in the chain representing a new mutation (Figure 14).

Dr Vogelstein's group studied inherited bowel cancer, a condition in which there are a number of recognized pre-cancerous (also called pre-malignant) steps that could be identified in patients. They collected tissues from patients and set about identifying which genes were abnormal in the various steps along the pathway from normal bowel lining to a clinically obvious cancer. It turned out to be possible to identify candidate genes that need to be damaged for each step of the cascade to occur. Subsequent work has demonstrated that similar cascades of events apply to all

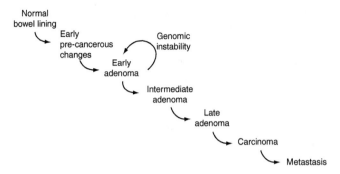

14. The Vogelstein cascade

tumour types, though the individual genes involved and the sequence of damage vary.

One fruitful way to identify genes has been to study families with so-called 'inherited' cancers. The term is a bit of a misnomer as the cancer is not inherited in the same way as, say, a diamond necklace, that is, as an intact, fully formed object. What is inherited is a greatly increased risk of developing a disease early, often in a very florid, aggressive form. One such disease is called adenomatous polyposis coli (APC). Patients with the disease develop multiple benign adenomas from an early age. In time, some of these progress to cancer, and without treatment death typically occurs in the early 40s from bowel cancer. Studies of patients with the disease showed that they had abnormalities in a particular gene, which was named APC. The identification of the APC gene in these patients led to further study of the function of the gene, which turns out to function as an 'off-switch'. If it is knocked out, an important check on cell growth is removed and adenomas form. As is often the way with inherited cancers, the much commoner, non-inherited cancers turned out to share similar abnormalities. Studies of non-inherited bowel cancer confirm that the APC gene is malfunctioning in around 80% of these sporadic cases, so the gene clearly has a key function in regulating the normal growth of the bowel lining.

Studies of inherited cancers thus often shed important light on the causation of the non-inherited counterpart disease. Study of these 'cancer families' helped identify key cancer-related genes such as APC, RB (linked to retinoblastoma, a rare childhood eye tumour), p53 (linked to Li-Fraumeni syndrome, in which patients develop multiple different cancers), and VHL (linked to von Hippel Lindau syndrome, a complex disorder that includes kidney cancer). In addition, examination of the varying natural history of the inherited disease helps us to understand what the normal function of these genes may be. All of the genes mentioned above are termed 'tumour-suppressor' genes, but this is a misnomer as this is not their primary role in the organism. As may be predicted from the APC gene, these genes are key regulators of the cell cycle (the first two aspects of the hallmarks mentioned above), and damage or deletion of function leads to uncontrolled growth. Examining the normal functions of these genes has shed important light on how the cell cycle is regulated. As lack of control of the cell cycle is a hallmark of cancer, many cancer treatments work by interfering with the cell cycle genes that are misfiring in the cancer cell. In addition, a new generation of cancer drugs, the targeted molecular therapies, is currently hitting the clinics and the news headlines (see Chapter 3). These drugs work by targeting specific molecules known to be misfiring in the cancer.

Not all inherited cancer genes are directly involved in the cell cycle, however. A good example is the VHL gene, originally identified in patients with von Hippel Lindau syndrome. Sufferers develop multiple abnormalities from an early age, including cysts in the nervous system, in particular the cerebellum (part of the brain involved in balance and coordination), spinal cord, and retina, together with kidney tumours both benign and malignant. The kidney tumours are typically bilateral, multiple, and occur from a young age. As for APC, the patient inherits one non-functioning gene; a single hit to the remaining gene leaves no functioning VHL protein in the cell. Given that renal tumours are relatively rare but are common in patients with VHL, this tells us that the chances of a given gene suffering one hit are relatively high, but suffering two hits takes much longer, hence sporadic tumours are single and have a much later age of onset.

Detailed study of the VHL gene has revealed that it is involved in sensing the oxygen levels in the cell. If oxygen is low, this leads to the production of signals to surrounding cells to start growing new blood vessels. In other words, it regulates angiogenesis, a key hallmark of cancer (see Figure 13). Further studies have shown that these changes are sufficient to drive the cancer cell in the test tube, and the replacement of the VHL gene in these models will reverse the cancerous characteristics of the cells. Furthermore, the kidney tumour type found in VHL patients, called renal cell carcinoma, is characteristically very rich in blood vessels, as may be predicted from the gene function. Study of sporadic (non-inherited) renal cell carcinomas has revealed that VHL is mutated in around 70% of cases, making the VHL/angiogenesis pathway an attractive target for therapy. Research into new VHL-based treatments for kidney cancer, a notoriously difficult cancer to treat once it has spread, has proved very fruitful, with six agents licensed since 2006 and several more pending for a disease for which only two agents had been licensed in the previous 25 years. All of these agents target aspects of the pathway identified by the genetic research summarized above.

Non-inherited cancer

While inherited cancers shed important light on the classes of genes involved in cancer, the majority of cases of cancer do not result from an obvious inherited predisposition. As we have seen in Chapter 1, the major causes of cancer death worldwide arise from tumours in the lung, stomach, liver, colon, and breast. Of these cancers, lung cancer is strongly linked to cigarette smoking, and liver cancer to infection with the hepatitis B virus, with a significant role for alcohol consumption. Cancers of the digestive tract are presumed to be linked to diet, but the precise causation is still poorly understood. Likewise, breast cancer (and prostate cancer in men) is clearly linked to both dietary and hormonal factors. How may these diverse influences act to produce the changes required to generate a cancer described above?

Lung cancer is the best understood example of how a carcinogen in the environment can interact to generate a cancer. The risk is clearly linked to amount of tobacco consumed – there is a dose effect – and the duration of consumption. Smokers who give up tobacco before getting cancer have a decreasing risk of developing the disease after stopping. In terms of a model like the Vogelstein cascade, smoking must be responsible for inducing the first steps of the cascade and continued smoking must also induce the subsequent steps. In older models of carcinogenesis, the initial step was often referred to as initiation and the subsequent steps as promotion of tumour growth, with a final step termed transformation. These terms still have value and in the laboratory, agents that convert non-malignant cell growths into cancerous ones are often referred to as transforming the cells. Analysis of tobacco smoke has revealed a host of agents that will result in transformation in cell culture systems. Detailed study of these smoke constituents has revealed the precise molecular mechanisms at work, down to the mode of interaction with the DNA double helix. One of the key culprits is called benzopyrene, and careful research has demonstrated it will bind to the DNA helix, damaging the structure. Figure 15 shows the benzopyrene molecule bound within a DNA double helix.

As mentioned above, there is clearly a need for DNA damage – an initiating event followed by a generally prolonged period of further damage accumulation, sometimes referred to as

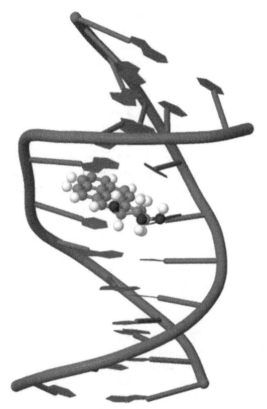

15. Benzopyrene bound within DNA

promotion – before a final transforming event turns the
pre-cancerous lesion into a full-blown cancer. In the case of
tobacco, the process appears to be driven by continuous
exposure to tobacco smoke, which has direct DNA-damaging
properties. For other diseases, in particular breast and prostate
cancers, the role of promoter is taken by the individual's own
hormones. As indicated in Chapter 1, risk of breast cancer is

influenced by duration of exposure of the breast to cyclical female hormones – hence early menarche and fewer pregnancies with no breast-feeding results in increased risk. The inference of this is that the continued cycles of changes in the breast induced by the menstrual cycle magnify any initial DNA damage done by some form of environmental carcinogen. A similar effect is seen in prostate cancer, in that men castrated early in life (for example, eunuchs) have a very low risk of prostate cancer compared to their peers who presumably are exposed to the same environmental carcinogens. A similar role is played by alcohol in liver disease. Alcohol, as already noted, is not a direct carcinogen – it will not damage DNA. However, heavy long-term abuse of alcohol induces cycles of damage and repair in the liver, with increased cell turnover. As with the cyclical changes in the breast, this continual increased activity serves to magnify the harm done by the DNA-damaging agents which must also be present, increasing the opportunity for accumulation of further DNA damage and the development of cancer.

As mentioned in Chapter 1, in the case of liver cancer, we also have detailed knowledge of the most frequent carcinogen – hepatitis B infection. The disease is a massive cause of suffering worldwide, but particularly in China and other parts of Asia where up to 10% of the population is chronically infected. There are lower rates in India and the Middle East, with rates less than 1% in Europe and North America. The risk of developing chronic infection is highest in those infected in infancy. Since 1982, a vaccine to HBV has been available. With vaccine programmes in place in various countries for some years, this has allowed scientists to complete the final test of the link between a virus and cancer – if the link were causal, preventing infection should and did prevent the disease. The precise molecular mechanism whereby the virus causes cancer is still being studied, but, as with smoking, the evidence for causation is now compelling.

Moving on to another cancer linked to infection – cervical cancer – we can see a similar story emerging. It was observed in the 1920s that cervical cancer was more common in women who had had high numbers of sexual partners, in particular prostitutes, and it was rare in nuns (except for those who had been previously sexually active), suggesting an infective, sexually transmitted cause. The disease was shown to be linked to infection with the human papillomavirus (HPV) by Harald Zur Hausen in 1976. Dr Zur Hausen found HPV DNA in both genital warts and cervical cancer. He received the Nobel Prize for Medicine for this discovery and his subsequent work in the field, which demonstrated the precise molecular links between the virus and the cancer. The virus produces various proteins which interact with two genes called Rb and p53, both key controllers of the cell cycle, providing an obvious route for generating a cancer.

The development of a vaccine against HPV and hence cervical cancer has proved more technically challenging than the HBV vaccine. However, the linkage between chronic viral infection and cancer allowed the study of the pre-malignant stages of cervical cancer. This led to the discovery that these could be identified in smears of cells taken with a wooden spatula from the cervix and then examined under the microscope. Identification of the pre-cancer stage, called cervical intra-epithelial neoplasia (CIN) or carcinoma-in-situ (CIS), allowed preventative treatment. Most European and North American countries have comprehensive screening based on the cervical smear test. These programmes have been estimated to have saved many thousands of lives. More recently, a vaccine against the varieties of HPV linked to cervical cancer became available in 2006 and is beginning to appear in public health vaccine programmes for girls as a way of preventing infection, with consequent reduction in cancer risk. There is some controversy about the vaccine as some interpret it as a way of protecting against the risks of promiscuity. However, protection against one sexually transmitted disease does not lower risks from others such as HIV. In addition, the vaccine will protect women against the risks of prior promiscuity in their partners, something they have no control over whatsoever. It will, however, take 10 to 20 years for this benefit to be seen, as this is the typical time lag between HPV infection and the development of cancer.

Chapter 3

How is cancer treated?

Cancer treatment is complex and typically will involve input from a number of different groups, ranging from a wide assortment of doctors, including general practitioners (family doctors), surgeons, oncologists, pathologists, radiologists, palliative care specialists, as well as a huge number of other trained personnel – nurses, radiographers, physiotherapists, technicians in laboratories and radiotherapy departments, theatre orderlies, the list goes on and on. The details of organization for these different groups vary enormously from country to country and are a function of both the politics and economics of healthcare.

To try and get around this problem, I will present the organization of cancer treatment as a journey from symptoms to diagnosis, treatment, follow-up, and palliative care for those experiencing incurable recurrence. Different healthcare systems will process these events in a variety of ways, but by and large, the underlying principles are pretty universal. The final part of the chapter gives an overview of the main different classes of treatment, such as surgery, chemotherapy, and radiotherapy.

Initial diagnosis and investigations

Most patients still present with symptoms such as a persistent cough or problems such as blood appearing in the urine. Significant numbers are also picked up by screening programmes, either organized on a systematic basis (for example, for breast and cervical cancer) or more informally (such as PSA testing for prostate cancer). Some cases are picked up as incidental findings in the course of investigation for some other problem. For example, an abdominal scan may detect an asymptomatic tumour in a kidney. I will return to these groups of patients later.

Most patients will present to their doctor with some sort of symptom they have noticed and which they are worried about. Although symptoms, like people, come in an unlimited number of varieties, they can mostly be grouped into those causing disruption of normal function, such as a brain tumour disrupting normal movement, or abnormal symptoms due to damage by the tumour, such as bleeding, pain, or cough. The period between initial symptoms and diagnosis of cancer may be very short or may sometimes run to years. Sometimes the delay in diagnosis is down to misinterpretation of symptoms by health professionals, sometimes deliberate self-neglect or self-deception by patients, and sometimes a mixture of the two.

Unsurprisingly, the perception that an opportunity to make an early diagnosis has been missed can cause severe subsequent problems in the relationship between the patient and their doctor, often at a time when they need them most. Family doctors have a tough time in this respect. For example, headache and backache are common symptoms, and in the vast majority of cases have benign causes that may need symptomatic remedies but do not need extensive investigation. Occasionally, of course, these symptoms may indicate an underlying brain or spinal tumour. Another example is the presence of blood in the bowel motions. All medical students know that this may indicate bowel cancer. All family doctors will know that for patients in the 'at risk' age range for bowel cancer, the presence of conditions like haemorrhoids (an irritating condition of the lower anus that can bleed) are virtually universal. How do they then set about distinguishing the banal from the severe (but rare) without grossly over-investigating their patients? The answer often lies in another basic skill taught in medical school – the art of taking an accurate history. Thus, a sudden and unexpected change such as severe bleeding mixed in with motions is much more likely to be due to a cancer than a small quantity of bright red blood being seen smeared on the toilet paper occurring over a period of years.

Screening for cancer

In an ideal world, we would be able to offer tests that picked up cancer before it reached the more serious stages, allowing early intervention and a much greater prospect of cure. Such a process is called screening and is now available for a number of cancers: breast, uterine, cervix, and bowel. In addition, the PSA blood test is a potential screening test for prostate cancer, but its use remains controversial. It is helpful to describe the characteristics of an ideal screening test and then examine how these tests shape up in practice.

This is illustrated in the following example:

Table 1 - features of an ideal screening test (Source: WHO)

- The target disease should be a common form of cancer, with high associated death rate
- Effective treatment, capable of reducing the risk of death if applied early enough, should be available
- Test procedures should be acceptable, safe, and relatively inexpensive

In addition, we need to consider:

- True positive rates: Sick people correctly diagnosed as sick
- False positive rates: Healthy people wrongly identified as sick
- True negative rates: Healthy people correctly identified as healthy
- False negative rates: Sick people wrongly identified as healthy

Table 2. Relation between results of liver scan and correct diagnosis

	Patients with the liver disease	Patients with no liver disease	Totals
Liver scan			
Abnormal (+)	231	32	263
Normal (-)	27	54	81
Totals	258	86	344

Thus the sensitivity (Patients with liver disease and abnormal scans/all patients with a positive scan) = 231/231+31 = 0.88

and the specificity (Patients with normal scans and no disease/all patients with normal scans) = 54/(27+54) = 0.67

A further measure is the positive predictive value (the proportion of patients with abnormal scans who have liver disease) = 231/(231+27) = 0.89

and the negative predictive value of a negative scan (the proportion of patients with normal scans who have no liver disease)

= 54/(32+86) = 0.45

For a test in the clinic, this is pretty good – a positive scan in someone suspected of having liver disease is a pretty good indicator that the person has the disease. How does this fare as a screening test, then?

To illustrate the difference between using a test for diagnosis in someone already known to be ill and screening for disease in people with no symptoms, we can look at the figures for breast cancer. Let us suppose that the rate of missed cases (the specificity) in those who we test is 10% and that the level of early, undetected disease is 1 in 500 people. If we now test 100,000 subjects, an ideal test would yield 200 positive tests in the cancer sufferers and 999,800 negative tests in those without the disease. However, our test, though good, is not perfect and will only detect 180 of the 200 cases, leaving 20 people wrongly reassured. Conversely, the test is also not completely specific. Let us say that 95% of those without the disease will test negative but 5% will wrongly test positive. When we apply this to our screening population, we see that this means that 5% of the 99,800 without the disease will falsely test positive. This works out as 4,999 false positive tests in people without the disease. This means that only a minority (180/4,999 = 4%) of those with a positive test actually have the disease, but 4,999 - 180 = 4,819 people have had a nasty scare. Furthermore, 20 have been falsely reassured and will go on to present with cancer anyway, possibly detected late as they may ignore the symptoms, believing themselves to be cancer-free. However, the overwhelming majority of those with a negative test (99,800 – more than 99%) really were free of the disease, so a negative test is pretty reassuring.

These worked examples are important, as they illustrate the limitations of screening tests which at first sight sound pretty good. In point of fact, the figures above are the *best* figures available – sensitivity and specificity fall in younger women (probably because their breast tissue is denser, making it harder to see abnormal lumps), leading to more incorrectly categorized cases. Furthermore, while the cost of the test itself is small, the cost of chasing up the false positives is much larger and needs to be factored into the costs of the screening programme.

There is a further problem when working out the benefit of screening. In our example above, we will identify cases of cancer earlier than would have happened without screening, potentially improving treatment prospects. However, with breast cancer, the cure rates are good, with three-quarters of diagnosed women being long-term survivors. This leaves the quarter who are destined to do badly, who are the main potential beneficiaries of screening. This is a relatively small number in relation to the numbers of tests carried out, and the downside is over-investigation of healthy women without breast cancer.

Investigating suspected cancer

Whether the patient has been picked up by a screening programme or has presented to their doctor with worrisome

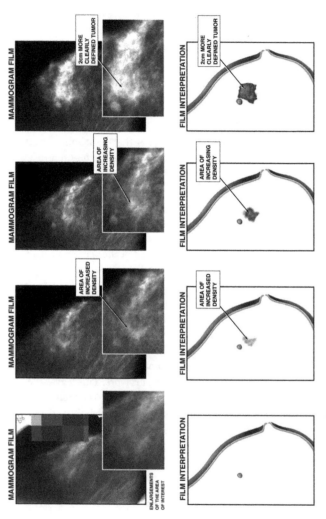

16. Mammogram of breast cancer

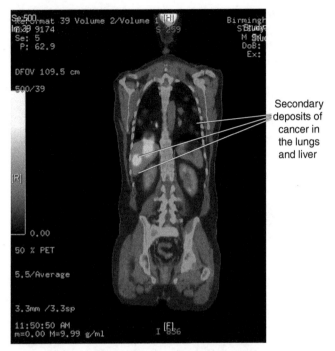

Secondary deposits of cancer in the lungs and liver

17. **Combined CT/PET (positron emission tomography) image of patient with advanced cancer with spread to lungs and liver**

symptoms, the next step is to carry out further tests to confirm or exclude the diagnosis. Diagnosis is usually based on a tissue sample (biopsy) of the affected organ, preceded by clinical examination by a doctor, imaging, and blood tests. Ideally, cancer would be investigated using non-invasive imaging tests. In practice, in almost all cases the diagnosis needs to be confirmed by examining a tissue sample in the laboratory. Imaging is key to deciding where and how to obtain tissue. Modern cross-sectional imaging either with X-rays – computed tomography, or CT, scans – or using magnetic resonance imaging (MRI) can give remarkably detailed pictures of internal organs and suspected tumours. However, even the best imaging is unable to show with certainty whether a mass is cancerous and also, even if the diagnosis of cancer is highly likely, exactly what sort of cancer. Occasionally the imaging is sufficient. For example, an elderly, frail, life-long heavy smoker with suspected lung cancer on a chest X-ray and who is unfit for any treatment may be spared the discomfort of a confirming biopsy. One or two other scenarios may also not require a biopsy – patients with extensive cancer deposits in bone (a common site of spread for prostate cancer) on imaging and a grossly elevated serum prostate specific antigen (PSA) can be reliably diagnosed as having widespread prostate cancer with no biopsy. The illustrations show specimen scans of a cancer in the breast (Figure 16) and secondary tumour deposits in the lung and liver (Figure 17). In all of these cases, the abnormalities are evident. However, even for radiologically obvious lesions such as these, a biopsy is generally required to determine the exact cancer type and hence the appropriate treatment.

The role of the pathologist in cancer diagnosis

The pathologist assesses small tissue samples taken, for example, via a needle – biopsies. Occasionally, for example in renal cancer, the initial material may be from a surgically removed organ, such as the diseased kidney. Mostly, this is done by mounting very thin slices of the removed tumour on slides and then carrying out a range of stains which highlight particular features of interest. The stained slides are then examined by the pathologist using a microscope. A commonly used stain is haematoxylin and eosin (usually called H&E) which highlights the various components of the cell such as the nucleus. Increasingly specialized stains are used which help further characterize the tumour. An example would be staining for the oestrogen receptor in breast cancer which helps predict the response of the cancer to both chemotherapy and hormone therapy. There are a rapidly growing number of available tests, mostly based on monoclonal antibodies (which are also increasing rapidly as a form of treatment – see below). In addition, tests can also be done to look for changes in the expression of particular genes or to look for the presence of particular mutations or rearrangements in chromosomes.

The primary question for the pathologist is: 'is it cancer?' If the answer is 'yes', then secondary questions include the specific type – in other words, in which organ did it start and which subtype. In addition, cancers are graded in terms of aggressiveness, typically on a scale of one (low) to three (high). Some cancers, for example prostate cancer, lymphoma (cancer of the lymph glands), and sarcomas (cancers of the connecting and structural tissues such as bone, muscle, or cartilage), have different grading systems, but the same principles apply. All of these systems are based on the size and shape of the cancer cells and how they compare to the normal cells in the organ in which they originated.

More recently, and increasingly, additional subclassification is based on molecular markers present on the cancer. These can be defined as characteristic features based on excessive levels of particular markers either in the tumour itself or circulating in blood (or sometimes present in urine). Probably the best-known example of a molecular marker is HER2 in breast cancer. This was initially described as a marker of poor outcome in breast and ovarian cancer by Dr Denis Slamon from UCLA in the late 1980s. This led to the development of the drug trastuzumab (Herceptin), intended to target cells with excessive amounts of the protein (termed over-expression). Landmark trials, initially in patients with advanced disease and subsequently in newly diagnosed patients, showed that the drug significantly improved outcomes for the 25% of women with tumours with high levels of the HER2 protein. Staining tumour samples for HER2 expression thus gives important information about prognosis (treatment outcomes) and also helps guide the choice of treatment.

The other major role for the pathologist in cancer care is the assessment of specimens resulting from surgical removal of organs containing cancer. In addition to the questions posed above, which will be reassessed with the larger specimen, the pathologist is also addressing issues such as:

- is the tumour confined to the organ that has been removed at surgery?
- are the surgical resection margins (the edges of the specimen) free of tumour?
- is there spread to other associated structures such as lymph glands?

Treatment decision-making

Having carried out a biopsy and appropriate imaging, a decision has to be made about the treatment approach for the patient. An important initial decision is whether or not cure is feasible. If treatment is going to be essentially palliative, this must be factored into decision-making – quality of life becomes paramount. If treatment is potentially curative, then different considerations apply – research has shown that patients will endure considerable side effects in return for a chance of cure. Whether the aim is cure, life prolongation, or palliation of symptoms, a range of approaches are available and may be used either alone or in combination. Decisions need to be reviewed on a regular basis and treatment adapted in accordance with side effects and tumour response – that is, whether or not things are improving.

Increasingly, in major healthcare systems, these decisions are not made by individual doctors but by a multi-disciplinary team, usually abbreviated to MDT (in the UK, this is now mandatory if the hospital is to receive reimbursement for cancer therapy). Typically, these teams will comprise surgeons, radiation and medical oncologists, radiologists, pathologists, and specialist nurses. The MDT will review the baseline information (termed staging information) prior to the consultation with the patient to review the various test results. Generally, these decisions will be based on national or international guidelines on best practice. The results and treatment options will then be discussed with the patient in the clinic, and the clinical plan finalized.

The various treatment modalities will be dealt with in turn, but before doing so, it may be helpful to give a broad breakdown of the relative importance of the treatment modalities. Figure 18 gives an estimate of how 100 'typical' patients would be treated in a modern Western healthcare system. Clearly, the numbers are for illustration only and will vary by country, and even within countries with local practice. For example, bladder cancer can be managed either by surgery to remove the bladder (cystectomy) or by radiotherapy to destroy the tumour, with surgery reserved for salvage of radiotherapy failures. In the USA, very few patients are managed electively with radiotherapy, which is reserved mostly for palliation (symptom control) in the elderly and frail. In contrast, in the UK, around two-thirds of patients are managed with primary radiotherapy, with surgery focused on the younger, fitter patients. These differences in practice stem largely from the differences in the

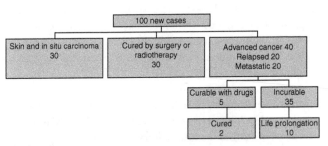

18. Distribution of cancer care between treatment modalities

UK and US health economies (see Chapter 5) rather than any evidence-driven differences.

The essential principle underlying the distribution is that around 30% of cases are only very locally invasive – for example, basal skin cancers (commonly called rodent ulcers) – and require a very limited local therapy, usually surgery but occasionally radiotherapy. Of the rest, around 40% of patients end up with widespread cancer and 30% have locally advanced cancer, which can be eradicated by local/regional treatments such as surgery or radiotherapy. As already indicated, the precise split varies in part by geography but also varies with anatomical site. For example, cancer of the colon is best treated with surgery rather than radiotherapy, as a normal large bowel is relatively intolerant of radiotherapy, and also targeting a mobile structure is clearly problematical. On the other hand, cancer of the uterine cervix (neck of the womb) is now predominantly treated by radiotherapy combined with simultaneous chemotherapy, with surgery reserved for salvage cases plus a limited role in assessing the disease for local spread.

Of the patients who end up with advanced cancer, around half present with this in the first place, the other half start out with apparently localized disease but then subsequently relapse with more widespread problems. Of patients who develop advanced (usually called metastatic) cancer, the majority will have essentially incurable disease. These will be diseases like advanced lung, bowel, breast, prostate, or liver cancer – the major cancer killers. A minority will have potentially chemocurable diseases such as testicular cancer, lymphoma, leukaemia, or certain childhood cancers.

It can be seen from this breakdown that the majority of patients cured of cancer in the 21st century are treated with modalities developed initially in the 19th century – surgery and radiotherapy. The major drug treatment advances, which drive so many of the news headlines, started in the mid-20th century and mostly extend lives in advanced disease rather than actually curing patients. This fact is well known to public health doctors but less well appreciated by the general public. It follows from this that in poorer economies, the maximum impact on cancer will be obtained by putting in place good basic surgery and radiotherapy. The best illustration of this is the survival rates worldwide for rectal cancer, for which the best results are obtained in Cuba, renowned for its well-organized medical care but with very limited access to the more expensive new drugs. Where resources are limited, cancer chemotherapy is best focused on the rare chemocurable cancers such as childhood leukaemia and testicular cancer. As these cancers mostly occur in younger people, the impact from drug spend in this area on life years saved is disproportionately high compared to spending on end-of-life cancer drugs in older patients. Drug therapy for advanced disease occurring in later life tends to have a much smaller impact on cure rates. Even if cures were common, the patients themselves are older and thus have more limited life expectancy anyway. This topic will be dealt with in more detail in Chapter 5.

Surgery

Surgery clearly dates back millennia, but the era of cancer surgery really dates back to the development of effective anaesthesia in the mid-19th century, which moved surgery from the ghastly, last-ditch 'gore-fest' of emergency amputations to controlled dissections. As already discussed, surgery to remove the tumour is one of the mainstays of cancer therapy (together with radiotherapy), and despite advances in drug treatment seems set to remain so for the foreseeable future. Increasingly, surgeons are developing minimally invasive (often called keyhole) techniques to operate without performing large incisions. These have the advantage of rapid postoperative recovery, but do increase operation times and are technically challenging. These techniques do allow older, frailer patients to be operated on due to the faster recovery times. They are also more generally attractive to all patient groups as they are less painful in the recovery period and rehabilitation to full normal function is quicker. Against this, operating via long metal tubes whilst peering down a modified telescope has been likened to tying your shoelaces with chopsticks, making exponents of open surgery claim that the key cancer outcomes – completeness of tumour

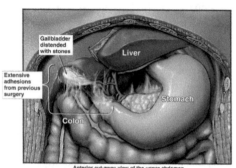

Anterior cut-away view of the upper abdomen

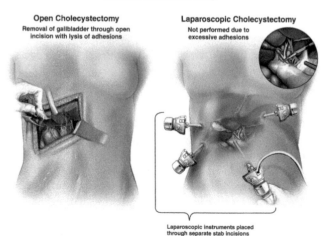

Open Cholecystectomy
Removal of gallbladder through open incision with lysis of adhesions

Laparoscopic Cholecystectomy
Not performed due to excessive adhesions

Laparoscopic instruments placed through separate stab incisions

19. Comparison of open and laparoscopic gall bladder removal

removal, for example – may be compromised. Assessment of this aspect of care is made by the pathologist – a key member of the cancer team.

A recent development in minimal access surgery is the robot-assisted procedure. In a robotic operation, the instruments are inserted manually and then fixed into the robot arms. Viewing ports are inserted and the surgeon operates at a console separate from the patient – essentially using computer games technology to manipulate the instruments remotely. There are potential downsides to this exciting technology – for example, the set-up time for the robot instruments is longer than directly manipulated 'keyhole' instruments. Also, the machines themselves cost around £1,000,000 to buy and approximately £150,000 per year to run. This is a considerable additional outlay over and above all the general infrastructure of operating theatres, wards, anaesthetic departments, and so on. Whether ultimately this will turn out to be both clinically and cost effective clearly remains to be seen. Certainly in the USA, there is now very strong consumer/patient

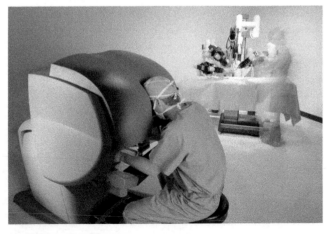

20. Robot-assisted surgery

demand for robotic surgery that may ultimately override the colder clinical considerations.

Radiotherapy

Radiotherapy is another 19th-century technology still going strong in the 21st century. Roentgen made the key observations underpinning modern radiotherapy in 1895 when he observed that invisible rays (which he called 'X-rays') were produced when electrons were fired at a target in a vacuum – revealed by their ability to blacken photographic film. It was rapidly realized that X-rays were transmitting energy and that this energy could be potentially focused for treatment as well as imaging. Within a matter of months, the first patients with skin tumours were treated – a breathtaking rate of innovation. The technologies of both imaging and therapy have gradually been refined and improved over the last century or so, and now form key components of modern cancer therapy. Indeed, as already noted, the most effective parts of modern cancer therapy remain surgery and radiotherapy, with the additional gain from drug treatment in terms of cure rates being relatively marginal. In wealthy first-world economies, drug treatments can clearly be funded over and above these two key planks of therapy. However, in poorer countries, where difficult choices have to be made, very few drugs offer good value for money in curative terms compared to surgery and radiotherapy.

After the initial observations of the effects of X-rays, either electrically generated or produced by using radioactive isotopes, the technology has been progressively refined. Initial technology based on the vacuum tubes described by Roentgen in the 19th century gave a beam which could penetrate to internal organs but which deposited considerably more of the dose nearer the skin. In the 1950s, much more powerful, so-called mega-voltage machines became available. These were based on the artificial isotope Cobalt-60, now superseded by an electrically based device called a linear accelerator, usually abbreviated to linac. These latter machines used the magnetron valve developed in the Second World War for radar. The pulsed energy can be used to 'shove' electrons into the target at much higher energies with much better properties for treating deep-seated tumours – a sort of electronic ploughshare from a high-tech sword.

Modern radiotherapy can be very precisely targeted by integrating treatment delivery with detailed imaging. Side effects arise in two ways. In structures such as skin, gut lining, and the mouth, the effects can be likened to sunburn, with severity depending on the dose received. Effects experienced depend on the site treated and may include diarrhoea with lower bowel treatment, or sore mouth, hair loss, and reddening in treated skin, and so on. A second group of side effects is experienced in solid structures such as lung and kidney. In these organs, there is little immediate effect, but if critical dose constraints are exceeded, the irradiated tissue will progressively fail. Dose to critical organs adjacent to the target tumour is thus a key restriction on the delivery of radiotherapy – a certain amount of toxicity will be worth accepting in order to treat the cancer, but clearly there comes a point when the damage may outweigh the benefit. Improved radiotherapy such as intensity-modulated radiotherapy (IMRT), involving very sophisticated dose distributions which appear to 'bend' dose around critical structures, is increasingly becoming available but increases costs and complexity of delivery. A linked development is on-board imaging in treatment machines which can be used to give image-guided radiotherapy (IGRT) where the treatment tracks movements in the tumour from day to day. The combination of IMRT and IGRT has the potential to both increase tumour control (by ensuring treatment is on target) and decrease side effects by better sparing of uninvolved tissues.

Hormone therapy

Although chemotherapy now dominates cancer drug therapy, it was a hormone-based drug therapy that was the first successful medicinal cancer treatment. Hormone therapy for cancer dates back to the 1940s following observations made by Charles Huggins, an American urologist, on patients with advanced prostate cancer.

The pioneers of hormone therapy reasoned that if the 'parent' tissue needed normal hormone levels, then the abnormal tumour derived from the tissue may retain this dependence. Trials of castration in advanced prostate cancer produced dramatic results, with rapid and substantial improvements in symptoms such as pain from cancer deposits in bone. Following this, administration of female hormones, which of course suppress male characteristics, was attempted, again with dramatic results. Sadly, these endocrine effects, while substantial, would last for only 1 or 2 years, the disease then recurring. Similar effects were observed in pre-menopausal women with breast cancer following removal of the ovaries. The subsequent decades have seen the development of a whole range of hormone-based medications for both prostate cancer and breast cancer in particular. One of these drugs, the oestrogen blocker tamoxifen, is probably responsible for saving more lives than any other anticancer drug. More than half a century on, new drugs targeting the hormone pathways are still appearing in the clinic.

Chemotherapy

If members of the public are asked to name the class of drugs most associated with cancer treatment, they will say chemotherapy. The term covers a wide range of different agents with diverse origins from antibiotics to plant extracts to synthetic chemicals based on DNA. All interfere with the mechanics of cell division and, as many tissues have dividing cells, this leads to the typical side effects such as nausea and vomiting (partly from damage to the gut lining, partly from a direct effect on the brain), hair loss (damage to hair follicles), and risk of infection (damage to the production of white blood cells needed to defend against infection). We are all familiar with the images of billiard-ball bald patients 'fighting' cancer (to use the tabloid press term). Whilst this does occur with chemotherapy, the reality is more varied, with much chemotherapy given in the outpatient setting producing little nausea or hair loss. Hair loss is hard to prevent, but it is not a uniform property of all chemotherapy drugs. Nausea and vomiting are now pretty largely preventable, allowing the administration of drugs hitherto considered too toxic, even to quite elderly patients. This is important because much chemotherapy is given for palliation of symptoms, hence quality of life is of paramount importance. There is arguably little point to life prolongation if the quality of that life is poor.

The first chemotherapy drugs were based on chemicals derived from mustard gas, used extensively to ghastly effect in the First World War. It was noted that soldiers exposed to these agents who survived would experience drops in their white blood cells (the cells in the blood that are responsible for defence against infection). There is, of course, a cancer of the white blood cells – usually termed leukaemia. Trials were carried out of mustard gas derivatives such as mustine in both leukaemia and a second related group of cancers called lymphoma. Patients in these trials experienced for the first time remissions of what had previously been untreatable conditions. With drugs used singly, unfortunately these remissions turned out to be temporary. However, further drugs followed, and trials established that using these drugs in combinations could lead to cures for patients with leukaemia and lymphoma.

A wave of new chemotherapy drugs followed, and in the 1970s and 1980s it was widely assumed that these would in turn lead to curative therapies for most cases of advanced cancer. These drugs came from a variety of sources. Plant extracts (vincristine, docetaxel, paclitaxel), complexed heavy metals (cisplatinum, carboplatin), and antibiotics (doxorubicin, mitomycin) proved to be fruitful areas of discovery leading to large-scale laboratory screening programmes looking for promising chemicals in a whole range of plant and bacterial extracts. Another area of discovery was compounds derived from the components of DNA or other building blocks of the cell division process, the best example being 5-fluoro-uracil, which is a derivative of uracil, one of the components of RNA (see Chapter 2). The extra fluorine atom in the molecule allows 5FU to interact with DNA and RNA but not to be processed normally – a molecular 'spanner' in the works.

In the 1970s and 1980s, further notable successes followed, in particular advanced testicular cancer was transformed from a lethal to a highly curable condition. The magnitude of this success is best illustrated by seven-times Tour de France champion Lance Armstrong who was diagnosed with very extensive disease, including brain involvement. After successful extensive chemotherapy, he went on to win his first Tour, followed by a record-breaking six further triumphs. Similar successes have been seen in the leukaemias and a range of childhood cancers. Sadly, however, the major cancer killers have proved to be more resistant to chemotherapy, with cures elusive, although most tumour types will respond to chemotherapy to a degree. It was suggested that the problem may have been that insufficiently large doses of chemotherapy were being given. However, a round of trials in the 1990s showed that even extreme doses of combination chemotherapy together with a bone marrow transplant were unable to cure major killers such as advanced breast cancer.

This realization has led to a change of emphasis. The observation that advanced disease, while incurable, would respond to chemotherapy for a while led to the testing of chemotherapy in the setting of early disease, as had previously been done with hormone therapy. It was known that many patients with no obvious disease nonetheless later developed recurrence. This suggested that there must be very small amounts of cancer lurking undetected. The hypothesis was that giving chemotherapy early may work better than waiting for detectable relapse. Initial trials were disappointing but with hindsight were simply too small to detect the benefits. When trial results were pooled in breast cancer, it was realized that there was a benefit to early chemotherapy, with women receiving it relapsing later and surviving longer compared to those for whom chemotherapy was saved as a 'salvage' treatment. This is called adjuvant therapy and works on the principle that so-called 'micro-metastatic' disease may be eradicable, whereas once the disease is visible on a scan it is incurable. Essentially, modern scanners, whilst very sensitive, are unable to detect tumours smaller than a few millimetres across. Hence we cannot distinguish between people who have been cured by initial surgery or radiotherapy and those who have apparently normal scans but in reality harbour small residual tumour deposits destined to cause relapse in the future. Subsequent studies have refined the drug combinations used and also the groups of women deriving most benefit. The problem with adjuvant therapy is that many women will do well just with surgery and radiotherapy, and thus derive no benefit from the chemotherapy, only toxicity and potential harm. This risk is greatest for those with lowest risk of disease recurrence, either due to less aggressive disease or high risk of death from other causes (for example, the very elderly).

More recently, greater emphasis has been placed on the role of chemotherapy in palliation of symptoms. This may seem like an oxymoron – giving toxic drugs to reduce suffering. However, improved symptom control, in particular with drugs that prevent the severe nausea previously associated with chemotherapy, has transformed the value of these agents for palliation. The survival gains seen are often relatively modest – typically a matter of months – leading to researchers developing methods for measuring quality of life. This allows comparison of toxic drugs producing benefit, for example by reducing pain, with alternatives often described under the blanket term of 'best supportive care' – painkillers, radiotherapy, and so on.

These two trends – adjuvant and palliative use – have greatly increased the cancer drug bill in the developed world (see Chapter 5) as, although the gains are relatively small, the numbers who can benefit are enormous, and this has resulted in widespread use of chemotherapy in relatively elderly cancer patients.

Monoclonal antibodies

Antibodies are a key component of the body's immune defences. Each antibody comprises a constant region and a variable region. The variable region is responsible for the binding of the antibody to its target – this is illustrated in Figure 21. The normal function of antibodies is to bind to invading infectious organisms – viruses, bacteria, and so on. When exposed to a new infection, the body's white blood cells identify it and select the cells (called lymphocytes) with the antibody-variable region best able to stick to and disable the invader. Production of the relevant cells is massively increased, followed by increased production of antibodies able to bind to the invader. Once bound, other immune cells identify the antibody-coated invaders and ingest them, using the antibody-constant region as a 'hook' for pulling them out of the circulation. The development of an immune system is one of the key evolutionary steps necessary for the existence of complex multicellular organisms. Those born with inherited defects in their immune systems struggle to survive childhood, underlining the importance of this function.

In the 1970s, technology was developed to exploit the ability of the immune system by manufacturing antibodies against 'artificial' targets such as cancer cells. These engineered targeted antibodies are called monoclonal antibodies – antibodies made by a single clone of cells – and can be made to stick to pretty much any chosen target. By picking targets on cancer cells, these natural molecules can be used both as an aid to imaging, by linkage to radioactive chemicals, or simply as treatments in their own right.

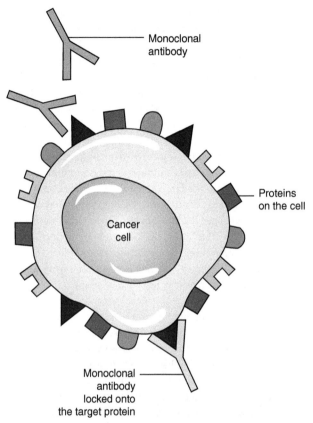

21. Diagram of a monoclonal antibody attached to a cancer cell

When they first appeared, it was thought that monoclonal antibodies would be the 'magic bullet' that would eradicate advanced cancer by being custom-made to order for each tumour. The reality sadly proved to be less dramatic, but 30 years on, monoclonal antibodies are now hitting the clinics in increasing numbers.

The best-known monoclonal antibody is probably trastuzumab, more often referred to by its trade name of Herceptin. The drug targets a protein on the surface of cancer cells known as HER2, part of a family of what are called growth factor receptors. These are best thought of as on/off switches regulated by circulating proteins (in this case called heregulin). Around one-third of breast cancers have an abnormal form of HER2 on the cell surface, essentially resulting in the switch being turned permanently 'on'. Breast tumours that are HER2-positive grow faster and more aggressively than those that are HER2-negative. Targeting HER2 on the cell surface thus seemed a logical strategy and monoclonal antibodies a good way of going about it. Initial studies were carried out in women with HER2-positive tumours and confirmed that the approach worked, with the drug being licensed in 2002. Although results were positive, with shrinkage of tumours seen, they were not as dramatic as may have been hoped for. Nonetheless, further trials were deemed worthwhile, this time using Herceptin in conjunction with chemotherapy for advanced disease. These trials produced more striking results, with women receiving Herceptin surviving around 50% longer than those receiving just chemotherapy.

The next stage of development proved to be even more interesting. Having shown benefit in incurable disease, the next step was to test the drug in patients with earlier disease at a potentially curable stage, a strategy that had already proved successful with hormone therapy and chemotherapy. The Herceptin adjuvant trials were an oncological triumph, with a halving of the relapse risk and the possibility that some of the previously incurable women were actually cured. There was a catch, however. Most women with early HER2-positive breast cancer actually already had a good outlook just with surgery, radiotherapy, and chemotherapy. If a woman is already cured by these treatments, she clearly cannot benefit from any further treatment (and may indeed be harmed, as Herceptin carries a risk of heart disease).

Conversely, some women will still die despite all current therapies, and therefore they too will benefit relatively little. In between are the real winners, converted from those destined to relapse to those potentially cured. This means that in the adjuvant (preventative) setting, the number needed who must be treated to benefit one of the real winners is high, maybe as many as 20. As the cost of Herceptin is substantial (around £30,000 per year), the effective cost per woman saved can be estimated as around 20 x 30,000 = £600,000. Unsurprisingly, therefore, when the drug was licensed for adjuvant use, a further storm of controversy followed – how much is it reasonable to spend to save one life?

Targeted molecular therapies

The DNA revolution and the sequencing of the entire human genome always promised that the benefits would result in better medicines. As more and more genes were cloned, it became possible to map the genes that were abnormal in cancer cells compared to normal cells. Once a key gene is identified, it then became possible to design drugs to target the abnormal gene or, more precisely, its associated protein product. One way to target therapies is with antibodies, as described above. The other way, now generating large numbers of new drugs, is to produce chemicals that interfere with the function, either of the abnormal protein itself or of one of the other elements of the same pathway in the cell. The first and probably best example of the first strategy is the leukaemia drug imatinib (Glivec). A form of leukaemia called chronic lymphocytic leukaemia (CLL) has long been known to be characterized by the presence of a so-called 'Philadelphia chromosome'. This abnormal chromosome is a fusion of two different chromosomes and results in the production of an abnormal protein derived from two different genes – called the bcr-abl fusion protein. Detailed molecular biology studies established that bcr-abl was both necessary and sufficient (the key conditions for a candidate new drug development) to drive the CLL cells, making it an ideal target. The drug imatinib was the first drug to successfully hit the target and it transformed the prognosis for CLL, with prolonged remissions occurring in patients resistant to the chemotherapy drugs previously used. Sadly, however, the remissions, while lengthy, were not permanent – the cancer cells eventually became resistant. This has been a feature of the targeted small molecular therapies – they are often exquisitely effective, with low side effects compared to chemotherapy, but generally do not lead to cures. However, as already noted in the chemotherapy section with leukaemia, initial use of these drugs singly also only produced remissions but not cures, so hopefully combination use will prove similarly beneficial. Time will tell.

The second approach to targeted therapy is to aim for the pathway that is linked to the 'core' abnormality. The best example of this is the recent transformation of kidney cancer therapy. Until recently, advanced kidney cancer was all but untreatable, with only two drugs licensed, interferon and interleukin-2, both of very limited effectiveness. Most kidney cancers occur 'spontaneously', that is to say, no other family members develop the same cancer. It had been observed many years ago that rare families developed the same tumours, often at a very young age – see the section in Chapter 2 on inherited cancer. One such inherited syndrome was described by von Hippel and Lindau and now bears their names. Patients with von Hippel Lindau (VHL) syndrome develop multiple early kidney cancers as part of the disease. Microscopically, the VHL cancers resembled the much more common, non-inherited cancers, so it was suspected that abnormalities in the VHL gene may be present in the spontaneous cancers, and this did indeed turn out to be the case. However, the problem in patients with VHL syndrome is that the normal function in the VHL protein is *missing*; hence targeting the VHL protein itself would only make the problem worse. Study of the VHL pathway revealed that as a result of VHL underactivity, proteins normally suppressed by the VHL protein became overactive. These include proteins driving the cells to divide and a further family of molecules driving the production of new blood vessels. Drugs were developed which targeted members of this pathway, either up- or downstream of the misfiring VHL protein, including three small molecular therapies, sunitinib, sorafenib, and temsirolimus, and a monoclonal antibody called bevacizumab.

Trials of these drugs have resulted in the treatment of advanced kidney cancer being revolutionized, with all four drugs licensed since 2006 and a further raft of additional drugs also heading into the clinic. As with CLL, however, although for the first time large advanced tumours could be made to shrink, the drugs do not result in cures in most cases, and treatment resistance develops with time. Trials are now focusing on adjuvant therapy, sequencing, and combinations in the hope that further survival gains can be made.

As with the Herceptin story above, the drugs have caused huge controversy due to their cost – patients need to be treated continuously rather than with a limited course of treatment, as was previously the norm with treatments such as chemotherapy. The drugs are expensive – around £25,000–£30,000 per year of treatment – with consequent variations in access (see Chapter 5). Unlike with Herceptin and breast cancer, however, purchasing authorities in a range of countries, including Canada, Australia, Scotland, and England, have been more resistant to funding treatments for a group of predominantly elderly male patients than they were for the very vocal women's breast cancer lobby.

Drugs used for symptom control

Although not directly treating the cancer, a range of supportive care drugs have contributed to big improvements in cancer treatments over the last 10 to 15 years. The improved anti-sickness drugs have already been mentioned. Also related to chemotherapy safety and delivery are the growth factors, in particular granulocyte colony stimulating factor (G-CSF) which boosts white blood cell counts, reducing infection risks. A second related product called GM-CSF (granulocyte-macrophage colony stimulating factor), initially developed for the same purpose, has turned out to have a valuable role in releasing blood cell precursors called stem cells into the circulation. This somewhat esoteric observation has allowed the harvesting of stem cells prior to high-dose chemotherapy intended to destroy the normal bone marrow. Previously patients needed a bone marrow transplant to 'rescue' them from such treatment, but it turns out that harvested stem cells do the same job but more quickly and with a much easier pre-treatment harvesting procedure, extending the range of patients suitable for these high-dose therapies.

Another area of recent research has been bone-protecting agents. Many cancers spread into bone with devastating consequences, including pain, fracture, and paralysis due to spinal column damage. Research demonstrated that the body 'over-reacting' to the cancer led, paradoxically, to increased damage. Drugs initially developed for osteoporosis (bone thinning) turned out to reduce this collateral, self-inflicted damage. The initial drugs available, such as clodronate, were relatively low in potency but later drugs, such as zoledronate and ibandronate, are many times more effective and can substantially reduce bone damage in patients with advanced cancer. Even more intriguingly, in adjuvant trials in high-risk breast cancer, zoledronate also appeared to reduce soft tissue disease, suggesting these agents may in addition have direct anticancer properties.

Conclusions

The improvements in cancer treatment seen in the last 100 years have been dramatic and have transformed the outcomes for millions of people across the world. Cancer treatment in the early 21st century is safer, more effective, and less toxic than it was 50 or 100 years ago. Surgery and radiotherapy continue to be refined and improved, with better targeting and minimal access technologies increasingly available. The ancillary imaging and pathology services will also continue to improve and allow better selection of treatment options in the future. The range of drugs and the effectiveness of those drugs are increasing rapidly, and this will generate further improvements in the coming years. The main problem with all this, as we shall see in Chapter 5, is the escalating cost, but grappling with this issue is better than not having the options available.

Chapter 4
Cancer research

Introduction

As we have already seen, the mainstays of cancer therapy remain surgery and radiotherapy, both of which date from the 19th century but which have undergone a process of continual technical improvement, which is still ongoing. Drug treatments for cancer are comparatively much more recent. The first successful cancer drug therapy was the use of synthetic female hormones to treat prostate cancer in the 1940s. Successful curative chemotherapy really dates from the 1970s with the development of treatments for leukaemias and lymphomas (cancers of the bone marrow and lymphatic system), although interestingly, the chemicals on which these treatments are based were previously developed for more nefarious purposes (as we have seen, mustine, one of the first successful drugs in this area, is based on the active ingredient of mustard gas). The development of new treatments and the improvement of existing ones clearly requires a process of research. This chapter will describe some of the ways in which research happens, in particular the differences between the rules for drugs and those for devices (such as radiotherapy machines) or techniques (surgery). These contrasts will be explored in some detail, as there are important differences, with significant anomalies resulting. The chapter will focus mostly on where new treatments come from, but similar trial structures apply to testing existing treatments against each other or for research into techniques of symptom control.

The development process for new surgical and radiotherapy techniques differs significantly from that applying to drugs. Typically, a surgical improvement will be a small technical change (for example, a better way to control bleeding) that does not fundamentally conceptually alter the underlying technique. Such improvements are often licensed essentially on a 'fitness for purpose' basis (that is, does it really help control bleeding?). Similar arguments apply to technical radiotherapy improvements (for example, better ways of targeting radiation to spare normal tissues). In general, it has been taken as self-evident that improvements of these sorts must be better and their implementation will follow. In fact, the improvements may be illusory and commercial pressure rather than any sound evidence base may drive their implementation. I will illustrate how and why this may arise using robotic surgical techniques and intensity-modulated radiotherapy as examples.

Drug treatments, on the other hand, have to meet fundamentally different criteria. Generally, an improvement in survival rates compared to the previous standard of care is required by regulatory authorities such as the Food and Drug Administration (FDA) in the USA. This means a new drug treatment requires testing in a series of clinical trials involving large numbers of patients. Broadly, these can be divided into three categories termed phases 1 to 3.

Phase 1 trials establish the safety and side-effect profile of a drug. Typically, these will involve small numbers of patients, for cancer drugs usually those who have run out of standard options and who will have had multiple previous treatments. Drugs with less dramatic effects, for example blood pressure drugs, will often be tested first on healthy volunteers. Phase 2 trials are larger and will often involve patients earlier in the 'cancer journey' than phase 1 studies, and they aim to confirm that a drug has useful activity against the target cancer. For a drug that looks promising, the final phase 3 trial will compare it with whatever is considered the standard of care. A phase 3 trial will involve many hundreds or even thousands of patients. There are a range of problems inherent in this design, ranging from consent and cost to legislative burdens. Phase 3 licensing trials are now almost always international affairs and have to comply with legislative frameworks from multiple countries, in particular the USA. The costs of such trials are enormous and explain the very high costs of new drugs – around $1 billion from synthesis to registration of a new cancer drug. The licensing process – which gives a company the lucrative right to market a drug or product – is tightly regulated by national or transnational bodies such as the FDA. This theme of regulation will be developed further in the next chapter – arguably, the high level of trial regulation protects the individual participant in a trial from possible harm at the expense of society at large by slowing the pace of improvement and driving up the costs of new drugs to the point when access is increasingly restricted, even in the most wealthy of economies.

Developing new cancer drugs

Basic science

Clearly, a massive body of biological research underpins cancer research. There have been huge advances made in the last 50 years, particularly the unravelling of the structure of DNA and the so-called 'central dogma' of biology – the relationship between DNA, RNA, and protein discussed in detail in Chapter 2. Previous generations of cancer drugs were developed largely by observing the effects of chemicals on cells, looking for drugs that were particularly effective at killing cancer cells. This research produced the chemotherapy drugs that appeared in large numbers in the 1970s and 1980s. Although new chemotherapy agents are still being produced, there is a sense of diminishing returns from more recent drugs compared to the huge advances of previous decades.

More recent research has focused on the evolving knowledge of the molecular signatures of cancer discussed in the previous chapter in relation to targeted small molecules and monoclonal antibodies. The human genome was sequenced in the late 20th century. The initial sequencing technology was cumbersome and slow, and the first complete sequence took many years to complete. Having completed this task, and with the overall structure of the human genome now known, it has become possible to sequence the genomes of specific cancers and to compare the cancer DNA to the patient's normal DNA extracted from their blood cells. This now takes teams in specialized laboratories a few weeks and costs are falling rapidly. The technology, time required, and costs are likely to improve dramatically over the next few years such that it will soon be possible to individually determine the DNA sequence of each patient's cancer as part of the diagnostic work-up. For the time being, this work is experimental, and remarkable results are emerging from this new field of study.

The human cell contains around 21,000 genes arranged in 23 chromosomes. Research comparing the DNA sequence of the entire 21,000 genes with the normal DNA of the patients has now been done for a number of cancers, and the results illustrate how small the line is between normal and cancerous cells. On average, experiments of this sort reveal abnormalities in around 40 to 60 genes. Put another way, if we picture the human genome as a library of 23 books (the chromosomes) each of around 1,000 pages (genes), there will be a total of 40 to 60 typographic errors in the entire cancer cell version of the 'library'. Furthermore, many of these genetic 'typos' will not actually alter the 'sense' of the gene – the protein produced will retain normal function. The number of key drivers of the cancer process boils down to around 12 pathways. The genes mutated or misfiring in cancers studied in this way all belong to one of these pathways and appear to be present in all cancers studied. This work points the way to the next stage of cancer drug development. The recent round of small molecules and monoclonals have largely (but not entirely) focused on single molecules such as HER2 being targeted by Herceptin. This recent whole genome work highlights the need to target pathways of multiple genes rather than single members. Drug screens in the future are likely to focus on this aspect of cancer biology, in tandem with whole genome screens to pinpoint the key mutated genes in particular cancers. It also opens the possibility that the drugs of tomorrow will be known to work in the presence of particular genetic signatures. Therefore, linking whole genome sequencing to diagnosis points the way to one of the 'holy grails' of cancer medicine – the personalized selection of drug therapies.

Pre-clinical phase

The first step in the development of new drugs is the identification of suitable compounds for study in human beings. Increasingly, this results from the sort of research work on cancer pathways described above. This search at present can take many forms, from screening of random compounds to the targeted synthesis of drugs to hit pre-specified abnormalities in the cancer cell. The drugs currently used in the clinic come from a range of sources, and some of these have been described in the previous chapter. The initial testing of a candidate drug will involve experiments with cancer cells in the laboratory. These cancer cells come from a variety of sources, ranging from human cancers to artificial tumours generated in laboratory animals. Some of the human cell lines were grown by taking fragments of a surgically removed cancer and placing it in cell culture medium in the laboratory. The process is conceptually attractive – you can test your drug on the 'real' cancer.

There are many such cell lines, possibly the most famous is the HeLa cell line. This was grown from a fragment of cervical cancer taken from a woman called Henrietta Lacks (also sometimes referred to as Helen Lane or Helen Larson in an attempt early on to preserve her privacy), and the cells are very widely used in laboratories around the world. Parenthetically, neither she nor her family gave their consent or permission for this process, resulting in a famous court case in California in 1990 in which it was decided that, in the USA, such a process was lawful. In the UK and other countries, the position is different and informed patient consent for tissue collection is now enforced by legislation. It has been calculated that so many HeLa cells have been cultured that they outnumber many times over the 'normal' cells produced by Ms Lacks in her lifetime, giving her a curious form of immortality. The problem with cell lines, however, is that most attempts to grow tumour cells from patients are unsuccessful. Hence the cell lines we have may be as unrepresentative of the typical cancer as HeLa cells are of the person that was Henrietta Lacks. Nonetheless, despite this limitation, human cancer cell lines remain a key component of cancer research and drug testing.

The second form of cell lines used are derived from animal tumours, mostly arising in mice. Many of these tumours are artificially engineered. A good example of this is an engineered cell line used in prostate cancer research. Mice do not get prostate cancer in the way that humans do. However, it is possible to identify genes that are expressed in mouse prostate and to use the promoter regions (see Chapter 2) of those genes to drive the production of proteins that cause cancer. In the case of mice, a gene with the curious name of 'large-T' from a cancer-causing virus called SV40 is used. Parenthetically, while many genes have names that are strings of unmemorable letters and numbers (there are 21,000 human genes alone after all – a lot to name), a subset have names varying from the odd (large-T) to the odder (hedgehog, notchless) to downright amusing – a pair of genes involved in cell signalling are called 'mad' and 'Max'!

In order to have mice develop prostate tumours, the hybrid gene containing the prostate specific gene promoter and the SV40-T gene must be inserted into a fertilized mouse egg. If the insertion is successful, a transgenic mouse results and the growing mice will now express the foreign gene in their prostate glands. As would be predicted, these mice go on to develop multiple prostate tumours. A number of these cancer-prone mice were bred, and the strain is called the TRansgenic Adenocarcinoma of the Mouse Prostate (TRAMP) model. These mice have proved useful in a number of ways. As the mice reliably develop tumours, they can be used to test cancer-preventing strategies such as dietary interventions. Secondly, the tumours can be used to test drug treatments for effectiveness. Thirdly, tumour cells arising in TRAMP mice have been successfully cultured in the lab and these cell lines can be used for experiments, either alone or re-implanted into adult animals from the same mouse strain – quicker and more reproducible than waiting for the tumours to develop in the TRAMP mice themselves. It is again obvious from the above discussions that such models are only representations of aspects of the human disease, not perfect replications of it. Hence, while useful, drugs must ultimately be tested in humans.

Before a drug can be administered to human subjects, a further phase of pre-clinical testing is required – toxicity testing. While animal models and cell culture provide valuable indications of whether a drug may be active in man, they do not tell us whether it is safe. We also need to know whether it is likely that we can achieve drug levels in patients that will be high enough to realistically have an impact on the cancer. The standard way of exploring this is to give escalating drug doses to groups of animals until we start to see animals dying from drug side effects. There are a number of rather grisly standard measures, such as the dose of drug that will kill a proportion of the test subjects – termed the lethal dose (LD) test. Measures such as LD50 (the dose that kills 50% of the animals) and LD10 (10% death rate) are widely used and attract much controversy from anti-vivisection groups. I don't propose to examine the ethics of animal testing *per se* – it seems to me to be something you believe is right or believe is wrong. If you fall in the latter category, then no amount of argument will generally alter opinions. I do believe it is worth critically examining the scientific basis of animal testing to try and minimize unnecessary suffering. There are many very obvious problems with LD50 testing – for example, the LD50 will vary widely for different species for a given compound and hence may still expose human subjects to risks. Nonetheless, compounds that turn out to be very toxic in LD50 tests at levels well below the necessary therapeutic levels are unlikely to be safe or worthwhile to test in humans. Whatever the rights and wrongs and limitations of pre-clinical toxicity testing, at present regulatory authorities require such testing on at least two species, one of which must be a non-rodent species such as the dog, before any human testing of a drug can begin.

Phase 1 trials

Having produced a candidate drug and completed the necessary pre-clinical testing package, the next step is testing in human subjects. Logically enough, this is termed a phase 1 trial. For many drugs, for example blood pressure pills, this testing will take place in 'normal', usually paid, volunteers. In general, these will be fit young men (not women, due to the risk of inadvertent damage to a foetus). For cancer drugs, which are often very toxic and frequently carcinogenic, this is clearly not an appropriate route, and phase 1 trials usually take place in patients who have exhausted standard treatment options. The classical phase 1 trial format is that the initial three patients are treated at a conservatively low dose and the effects observed. If no unacceptable toxicity occurs, then a further three patients will be treated at a higher dose, and so on. Clearly, for most drugs, eventually a dose level will be reached at which unacceptable side effects occur (termed 'dose-limiting toxicity', or DLT). If a patient experiences a DLT, additional patients are treated at the same dose level. If two or more out of six experience a DLT, then the 'maximum tolerated dose' (MTD) for the drug is reached and the trial ends. The dose level below the MTD will be used for further study.

The classical phase 1 trial has the merit of simplicity, but there are clearly limitations as well. Firstly, different patients will have varying susceptibility to potentially dose-limiting side effects. If the trial includes too many side-effect-prone patients, the estimated maximum tolerated dose will be too low, and vice versa. Secondly, not all drugs need to be used at the maximum tolerated dose. For example, a drug blocking a hormone receptor only needs to be given in sufficient quantity to block the target. Any additional drug given above this level is only adding toxicity with no benefit. For trials with drugs of this sort, it is therefore important to specify the endpoint required to avoid unnecessary drug exposure to participants.

The main problem with phase 1 trials relates to the needs of the patients. Mostly, these studies are happening in patients who have exhausted all standard therapy options and who are clearly desperate for further viable therapies. By its very nature, the phase 1 trial is mostly delivering drug below the likely therapeutic range with a consequent low chance of benefit. Furthermore, at least two of the last six patients entered in a study will receive too high a dose and will experience a high level of side effects. Finally, most drugs entering phase 1 will actually turn out to be of little therapeutic value due to either unforeseen problems preventing delivery of sufficient drug or simply a lack of efficacy against the target cancers. For most patients, therefore, entering a phase 1 trial needs to be seen largely as an act of altruism, and it is indeed true that many patients entering trials will say things like 'well if it helps people after me, it will be worth it'. Nonetheless, ethics committees and doctors must be careful to protect vulnerable and desperate patients from harm in these trials.

Phase 2

If an agent performs well in phase 1 – in other words, side effects are manageable and acceptable, usually with some evidence of a positive effect on the cancer, then a phase 2 trial will follow. The aim of phase 2 studies is to study the efficacy of the drug in more detail. The drug will be tested at the optimal dose defined in phase 1 in a group of patients assessed as likely to benefit from the drug. This is clearly different to phase 1 as the risk of under- or overdosing is much reduced, though it still remains, due to the limitations of the dose-finding mechanisms in phase 1 discussed above. Furthermore, as the patients are selected on the basis of likely benefit, the risk/benefit ratio for participants is much better. Typically, up to 40 or 50 patients will enter a phase 2 trial, and the endpoints will be efficacy, and of course safety, in the more defined, usually somewhat fitter, patient population.

Defining efficacy is a major problem. Generally, agents that produce tumour shrinkage are defined as active, and this has led to standardized ways of defining how much shrinkage constitutes a worthwhile response. The most widely used method is the RECIST (Response Evaluation Criteria In Solid Tumors) system, first published in 2000 and updated in January 2009. Disease responses are broadly classified as follows:

- complete response: all assessable disease disappeared;
- partial response: reduction in size by pre-specified amount of all assessable disease;
- stable disease: insufficient change to be put in another category;
- progressive disease: worsening of disease by pre-specified amount or appearance of new cancer deposits.

The principle underlying this system of assessment is simple; the application in practice is complex. As with many things, the devil is in the detail – the following is a list of tricky issues (not comprehensive) to illustrate the difficulties:

- How much should a tumour grow before it counts as progression?
- How much should it shrink to count as a response to treatment?
- What if some lumps shrink but not others?
- When should you carry out the response measurements (too early and you may under-report; too late and patients may have started relapsing)?

to obtain a licence. The comparator may be an existing drug or combination of drugs, or it may be what is termed 'best supportive care'. This latter option is chosen when there is no clear-cut standard therapy – patients receive whichever palliative measures the clinician thinks appropriate.

The hallmark feature of phase 3 trials is that the patients are randomly assigned between the treatment options. This ensures that patients will be evenly distributed between the various arms of the trial and minimizes the risk of differences in outcomes arising due to patients with a better or worse prognosis being concentrated in one arm of the trial. Whilst the design makes good scientific sense and is regarded as the 'gold standard' method of assessment, as always there are limitations.

Firstly and most obviously, where the control arm is best supportive care or worse still a placebo medication, there is understandable reluctance on the part of patients. Careful explanation and support is clearly required, particularly to make the point that if there is no other proven alternative, then treatment outside the trial will be no different to the control arm. Often, however, a phase 3 trial is not comparing the new drug with placebo but with the current standard therapy. This is generally a much easier discussion in the clinic as everyone receives treatment and the new medicine may be less good than the old one – we don't know until we do the trial. Even if the control is placebo, it is by no means a given that the new drug will turn out better – there are plenty of examples of trials in which the drug was no better than placebo, and even examples when the drug was worse – the drug was both toxic and ineffective.

Secondly, most new medicines will be only a little better than the existing ones, hence the likely differences between the trial arms will be small. In order to detect small differences, large sample sizes are necessary to ensure statistical confidence in the outcomes. Statistics is a much mocked, maligned, and misunderstood science, so it is helpful to illustrate why sample sizes need to be big with a simple example. Suppose we want to assess whether a coin used for a coin toss is evenly balanced or biased to either heads or tails. If we toss once, then we get either heads or tails (ignoring the possibility that the coin balances on its edge!). If we toss again and get the same, we have (say) 100% heads, 0% tails. No one would say the coin was biased on this size of sample, though. Suppose we carry on and get to 10 tosses – 6 heads, 4 tails – would we be confident that the coin was biased? Probably not. However, if we get to 100 tosses with 60 heads and 40 tails, or 1,000 tosses with 600 heads and 400 tails, we would have increasing confidence that the coin was indeed biased. The reverse of the problem is more difficult: if we got 501 versus 499, would we say the coin was biased? Again, probably not, but how about 510 versus 490? 520 versus 480? How similar can the numbers be in order that the difference is probably by chance rather than due to a biased coin? Even a big difference like 600 versus 400 can occur by chance with an unbiased coin, but would be very unlikely. The statistics plan for a trial is therefore key and will specify how many patients will be needed to reliably detect the minimum difference deemed to be clinically important in advance of the trial starting. For a trial testing a new drug in advanced cancer, this will be along the lines of an average improvement in survival of at least three months. As with our coin flip, this could arise by chance so the trial statistician will calculate how many patients are needed to show (or exclude) this difference reliably – usually defined (largely arbitrarily) as the chance result occurring fewer than 1 in 20 times.

For most modern trials, there will be a committee (usually called the Independent Data Monitoring Committee, IDMC, or Data and Safety Monitoring Committee, DSMC) set up to independently monitor the results as they accrue. This is in place to protect patients primarily – if there are unforeseen toxicity problems, for example, the trial may be stopped early. Later on in the trial, the IDMC can end the study if the predefined endpoints are met early.

This allows early dissemination of the data and allows other patients access to the drug earlier. Conversely, the IDMC can also determine that the trial is never likely to show significant differences and stop the trial early on grounds of futility.

Endpoints in trials are controversial. Trials are expensive, often $100 million plus, and hence drug companies want them to be as small and quick as possible. Conversely, regulators want the most reliable outcome measures and hence longer follow-up periods or larger sample sizes. Society at large has needs somewhere in between. We all want better medicines, and if we've got cancer, we want them now. Equally, we want them to be safe. Also, the larger and longer the trial, the more the drug company has to charge for the drug in order to pay back the higher development costs – see Chapter 5 for a more detailed discussion of this issue. As health budgets grow, so pressure to reduce drug costs rises, making availability of new drugs increasingly restricted for cancer patients in poorer economies. As a way out of these conflicting tensions, increasingly, researchers are looking for what are called 'surrogate' endpoints. The aim is to pick an early endpoint that will accurately predict the final outcome of the trial. The response rate in a phase 2 trial is an example of a surrogate endpoint used to select a drug for phase 3 study. The problem is that the correlation between response rate and the sort of endpoints regulators require, such as improved survival, is not sufficiently good to allow a high response rate in phase 2 to lead directly to a licence. The same will generally apply to comparisons of the response rates in randomized trials.

In order to get away from using survival-based comparisons, which clearly take a long time, investigators must show that some earlier measure reliably predicts the final outcome. An example of such a measure is the 'time to progression' mentioned above. This is the time taken for the tumour to grow or spread by pre-specified amounts and is commonly used as a registration trial endpoint in early breast cancer. In some disease settings, for example, PSA in prostate cancer, the candidate marker is unreliable, and drugs in prostate cancer are still currently stuck with needing to show improved survival to get a licence. In prostate cancer, studies are currently evaluating a novel method of response which is counting the number of circulating tumour cells. Typically, these are present in tiny numbers – around 5 per 7.5 millilitres of blood is the key cut-off level – a very tiny number of needles in a massive haystack of tens of millions of blood cells. If validated, such a test could greatly accelerate the pace of cancer drug development in diseases like prostate cancer currently stuck with overall survival endpoints. As shorter trials are cheaper, it could also reduce the price of the drug when licensed.

Comparisons of existing treatments

The phase 1–3 schema described above can broadly be fitted to any new technique or drug combination, however requirements differ in different countries. Trials comparing existing drugs in novel combinations are often undertaken by academic organizations such as Cancer Research UK or the US National Cancer Institute. Using the template above will give reliable results that can influence practice and are the gold standard for advancing medical practice in general. The system becomes much less clear with surgical techniques, radiotherapy equipment, other devices, and biomarkers, though. For example, new technologies such as robotic surgery are introduced as incremental improvements. These 'improvements' are treated as self-evident, when in fact they may be nothing of the sort. For example, comparing open with robot-assisted surgery: access routes to the body are different; the tactile connection between the surgeon's hands and the tissues is lost in robot-assisted surgery; control of bleeding or complications such as bowel perforation may present different risks, possibly requiring conversion from robot-assisted to an open conventional operation; theatre times may be longer when surgeons are training, and so on. It is clearly entirely plausible that each of these factors may substantially affect outcomes. In addition, there is the massive issue of cost. A surgical robot costs over £1 million, with another £100,000–£150,000 annual running costs. Even if the outcomes are better, how much is it worth paying for, say, earlier discharge from hospital?

One might expect that the introduction of such a technique, for example for prostate removal, would require the same sort of trials that new drugs for prostate cancer require, with equivalence or better in outcomes. No such trial has ever been carried out, yet surgical robots are working in major surgical centres across the world, particularly in the USA. Why the massive discrepancy? In essence, new devices simply have to demonstrate safety and fitness for the purpose for which they are designed. Where changes are genuinely small and incremental clearly a massive trial to show that a new scalpel is slightly better would be impractical and probably meaningless. At some point, the change ceases to be incremental and surgical robots seem to me to be a good example of this, yet are still treated as if they were simply a slightly better scalpel. In the USA in particular, buying a surgical robot has become an essential part of the marketing of a hospital – it is an iconic piece of kit – what go-ahead institution would want to be without one? Grappling with this issue is likely to become more and more important as healthcare systems struggle with rising costs. Conceivably, of course, new technologies may actually save costs. Sticking with the robots, it is not implausible that the claimed shorter learning curve, shorter hospital stay, and reduced complication rates could pay back the capital and running costs. At present, however, we simply don't know.

Similar arguments apply to tests such as imaging and other diagnostic tests. Again, there is an element of not needing to do research to validate the obvious – a scan with a sharper image is likely to be better than a fuzzy one! However, when we look more closely, things get more tricky. For example, one of the key drivers to decision-making is whether the cancer has spread to a particular organ. In general, if a scan looks abnormal in a particular area known to be at risk, it is likely that this represents disease. The

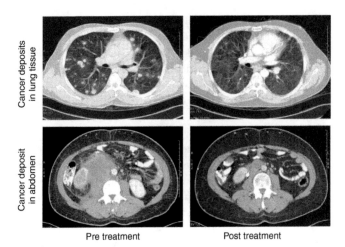

Cancer deposits in lung tissue		
Cancer deposit in abdomen		

Pre treatment   Post treatment

22. Examples of tumour responses on scans

converse is not the case, however – a negative scan could be negative or could mean the disease is below the threshold for detection. This is illustrated by the hypothetical liver scan discussed in Chapter 3. A good example of this sort of problem is the detection of cancer in lymph nodes. As lymph nodes are normal structures and cancer in lymph nodes is of similar density (and therefore imaging appearance) to the normal tissue, imaging can only tell us if nodes are of normal or abnormal dimensions – typically, the cut-off size is around 5 millimetres. Clearly, if we have a 4-millimetre cancer deposit replacing the bulk of a node, it will therefore look 'normal'.

Suppose a potentially better imaging test for node disease is developed, how should it be evaluated? Such a test would fall into the same sort of regulatory route as surgical devices – we need to show safety and fitness for purpose. Safety is straightforward – the phase 1/2 route clearly works fine, but how do we demonstrate 'fitness for purpose'? The answer is some form of clinical trial, but the question of endpoints is very tricky – how many 'normal' lymph nodes harbouring small cancers do we need to detect to be worthwhile? How many are we allowed to miss? How do we evaluate the 'true' positive and negative rates? Should we move to broader clinical outcomes rather than counting lymph nodes – for example, does the application of the test result in better clinical results, for example longer survival times, than the standard way of managing the patient?

These are all very difficult issues when applied to imaging technology when the acquisition costs of new scanners are very high. Even for technologies that augment existing scanners, for example new contrast medium drugs, the issues are substantial, and there is not a single consistent route across the globe.

Similar arguments apply to diagnostic tests. Again, at first sight, the problem would seem simple – if we have a blood test that correlates with the cancer, then we should use it as part of the basis for clinical decisions. However, if we examine the literature, we find many examples of tests that correlate with presence or absence of disease but very few are actually used clinically – why should this be? The principal answer to this is that the test has to give additional information over what we know already. For example, there are a whole range of urine tests that correlate with the presence of bladder cancer but none are used in the UK. Patients with suspected bladder cancer need a cystoscopy to confirm the diagnosis. The available urine tests are not reliable enough to exclude patients from a cystoscopy. Once the bladder has been examined, if a tumour is seen, a biopsy is needed. Again, the tests are not sufficiently reliable to obviate the need for biopsy. In addition, the excision biopsy is also part of the treatment, so however good the test, the patient still needs the operation. How about predicting prognosis? Again, the urine test is good but not as good as the pathological study of the removed tumour, so again it adds nothing. Given the above, the correct test for a diagnostic procedure is its effect on outcomes – can the test spare invasive procedures or predict which of a range of treatment options is best? This requires large-scale trials similar to those needed to license a drug and is the reason there are so few established tests or markers used in the clinic as decision aids.

There are examples of markers that correlate well with the disease and can be used to predict clinical events in advance of clinical symptoms or obvious scan changes. Examples of such markers include PSA in prostate cancer, CA125 in ovarian cancer, and AFP and HCG in testicular cancer. Even when good markers exist, they cannot necessarily replace other clinical methods of assessment. For example, while changes in PSA largely reflect changes in disease status, some treatments that affect the clinical outcomes (the bone-hardening drugs called bisphosphonates are a good example) have very little effect on PSA levels despite helping prevent bone damage by the cancer. Even more surprisingly, a recent huge study in ovarian cancer and the use of markers produced very counter-intuitive results. A rising level of CA125 in the blood accurately predicts clinical relapse. One might expect that treating relapse early would be better than waiting until symptoms developed. The study compared a policy of marker-driven treatment (that is, treatment for relapse started with rising marker levels) with clinical symptom-driven treatment. A total of around 1,500 women took part in the study, and the earlier introduction of treatment in women with more intensive monitoring did not affect survival times. Even more surprisingly, quality of life and anxiety levels were better in the women with the clinically driven treatment – tighter monitoring and earlier treatment were actually therefore inferior overall.

A huge focus of current research is individualized therapy – identifying markers that allow treatment to be tailored to the individual. There are many ways tumours can be characterized – by their DNA mutations, by their patterns of protein expression, by looking at the activities of different enzymes. However, while it is relatively easy to identify patterns that correlate with different outcomes, it will be obvious from the above discussion that this will not be sufficient to allow treatment to be altered. To demonstrate clinical value will require clinical trials comparing the candidate marker-driven policy with standard care. As the ovarian cancer example above shows, even having a good marker does not guarantee the expected result. A further problem that may emerge is that the numbers of candidate markers being developed may exceed the capacity of research teams to carry out trials, possibly many times over. Furthermore, markers effectively change a disease from being a homogenous entity to a number of distinct subentities. As good trials need large numbers, this makes doing trials more difficult – the disease effectively becomes rarer. This is illustrated by recent changes in renal cancer. A number of pathological variants had been described some time ago but until the advent of targeted small molecules, this made no difference to treatment options. As already discussed, the abnormalities in clear cell renal cancer (around 70% of the total) lead to new treatments. What then for the remaining 30%? Several different further subtypes make up this 30%, hence trials now become difficult as each is really rather uncommon. As a result, we don't really know how to manage these subgroups. These so-called 'orphan' diseases will become increasingly common and problematical as there will be little in the way of trial data to inform treatments, and trials will be difficult due to lack of numbers.

Conclusions

The coming years will see many exciting developments in new cancer drugs, new biomarkers, and exciting and futuristic technology such as surgical robots. How we incorporate these developments in practice will depend in large measure on clinical research to underpin their use. However, new technologies in particular will have a tendency to be introduced via the marketing rather than trials route. How we license, regulate, and fund these devices will become increasingly problematical as healthcare budgets come under pressure with an ageing population and the massive debt overhang of the credit crunch.

Chapter 5
The economics of cancer care

The previous chapters have illustrated the highly complex nature of modern cancer care and the rapid rate of change in both medical technology and drug therapy. These changes are underpinned by extensive investment in new treatments by both drug and medical equipment manufacturers, as illustrated in the previous chapter. Clearly, new treatments must be paid for and in general will cost more than the older technologies they replace. There are exceptions to this – for example, a treatment that improved the cure rate could reduce downstream expenditure on subsequent therapies and so may result in a net decrease in healthcare resource use. Measuring these interdependent changes is clearly complex, hence a lot of healthcare economic decision-making is focused on the direct acquisition costs of the new technology (which are easy to measure) rather than secondary downstream changes. Frequently with cancer care, these costs are focused near the end of life and result in contentious funding dilemmas. How these dilemmas are dealt with by different healthcare systems forms part of this chapter.

Economics also impinges on cancer care at a more macro-economic level than the cost of an individual drug. In general, the developed economies of the world have comprehensive healthcare systems that broadly cover health issues from cradle to grave. Different systems have different pros and cons, but the major difference is between the developed and less developed world. Clearly, if basic infrastructure is lacking, whether or not to buy an expensive new drug is not a relevant discussion for most of the population. It is possible to estimate the size of these effects: Figure 23 shows the interaction between per capita gross national product (pcGNP) and life expectancy in years. As can be seen, there are some countries with very low income and as would be expected, low life expectancy. However, there are others with pcGNP of less than $1,000 per year but where life expectancy exceeds 65 years. These countries include places like Egypt, Trinidad, and China. Common features of these countries are an integrated public health system and good perinatal care. Conversely, there are countries with pcGNP of more than $2,000 with life expectancy of less than 60 years. The problem here appears to be high levels of HIV infection. Thus in broad terms, how rich a country is will affect, not surprisingly, the quality of healthcare and life expectancy, but also other factors play an important part. Some of these factors can be readily influenced by factors within the control of governments – overall organization to get maximum impact from resources, public health campaigns, and so on. Conversely, at the upper end of the spectrum, once a certain level of national income is reached, there is very little further gain possible, with an apparent ceiling of life expectancy in the high 70s. Whether this will change in the future with improving technology remains to be seen.

If we move on to examine the effects of national income on cancer, we see another interesting effect. As wealth increases, so does the risk of developing cancer. This is partly an effect of lengthening life expectancy – if you don't starve or die young from infection, you have a much better chance of living to relative old age and getting cancer. Other factors are also at play: for example, once national income exceeds around $5,000 per person, cancer occurs at a rate of 250–400 cases per 100,000 people per year – see Figure 24. However, there are a number of countries with income

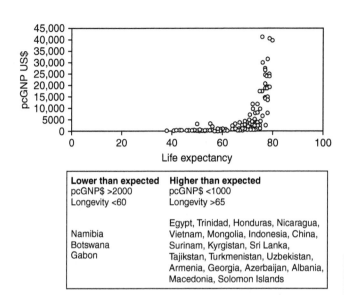

Lower than expected pcGNP\$ >2000 Longevity <60	Higher than expected pcGNP\$ <1000 Longevity >65
Namibia Botswana Gabon	Egypt, Trinidad, Honduras, Nicaragua, Vietnam, Mongolia, Indonesia, China, Surinam, Kyrgistan, Sri Lanka, Tajikstan, Turkmenistan, Uzbekistan, Armenia, Georgia, Azerbaijan, Albania, Macedonia, Solomon Islands

23. **National income per person and life expectancy**

in this bracket but with a cancer rate of less than one-third of this rate, all in the Middle East. This has been attributed to widespread adherence to more traditional, less Westernized lifestyles despite rising national income. Conversely, there is a cluster of countries with Western-style high cancer rates but income of less than \$5,000 per head. These turn out to be former Soviet bloc states who seem at first glance to have the worst of outcomes – Western diseases at developing world incomes. On closer inspection, however, the picture is less gloomy – the low income is real but the high cancer rates reflect long life expectancy due to well-organized healthcare systems. The recent discussions about the relative merits of 'socialized medicine', and in particular the NHS and the US system, highlight the need for dispassionate analysis. Whilst it is true that there are differences in some outcomes between the US and UK, overall life expectancy is very

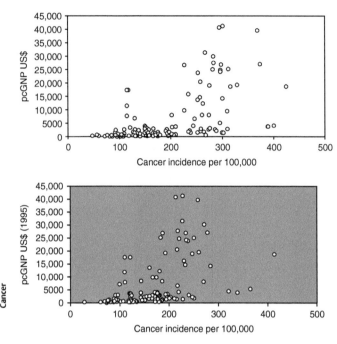

24. National income per person and cancer risk, for men (above) and for women (below)

similar for all countries with well-developed healthcare systems –
despite recent US Republican talk of NHS 'death panels', the truth
is that Western healthcare is pretty good at keeping most of its
citizens alive into old age.

Whilst all of this is true at the level of state funding, when cancer
therapy tends to hit the press is when access to a new therapy is
denied someone, usually presented as a variant of the staple news
story of 'patient refused life-saving drug by faceless bureaucrat'.
This is the origin of the Republican allegations about NHS death

panels (in truth, of course, US patients with no healthcare will also be denied the same treatment by a different set of bureaucrats or perhaps their bank manager). Why do these stories occur in some of the wealthiest countries in the world? What are the likely future trends in funding and costs?

Like most commodities, medical care tends to cost more year on year – inflation. It is possible to measure the rate of medical inflation, and in general this turns out to be higher than the underlying inflation rate in the economy. This is important as it means that without cost-cutting, healthcare over time will consume a bigger proportion of national income in keeping up with new technologies. This is best illustrated by the US economy where the medical inflation rate in 2008 was 6.9% – roughly double the rest of the economy. On current projections, this would see the US health spend increase from 17% of national income in 2008 to 20% by 2017. The massive changes in the world economy since the banking crisis make it very unlikely that this can be sustained. Similar figures apply in all the major economies. Why are costs rising in this fashion? After all, when the NHS was set up, Aneurin Bevin, one of its key architects, envisaged falling costs with time as health improved. The reason lies in the costs of developing new treatments. A licensing trial for a cancer treatment will typically cost around £100,000,000. Newly licensed drugs thus need to recoup these massive development costs, plus the costs of all the drugs that fell by the wayside in the process and will thus never generate any revenue. Patent life remaining by the time a drug is licensed is typically 10 years or less, as drugs need to be patent-protected many years before the licensing process is complete. The bulk of the cost of a new drug therefore reflects the costs incurred before licence – the actual manufacturing, while expensive, is typically only a small proportion of the price per pill. When a drug comes off patent the cost of a drug will usually fall with generic competition by around 90–95%, reflecting this.

The price charged for a new drug will thus be geared to paying back the massive development costs and then turning a profit before the patent licence expires. With globalization, prices tend to be similar worldwide, making new drugs particularly hard to afford in poorer countries. The pricing policies of pharmaceutical companies are not in the public domain but are presumably set to maximize income worldwide. For some countries, such as the UK, Australia, and New Zealand, this will often be above the price the health system is prepared to pay. This is presumably offset by the higher income generated by the greater price obtained in less restrictive health systems. For example, in France, once a drug is licensed, it can be freely prescribed by the relevant specialist with no direct expenditure cap. This has a big influence on rates of uptake and total spend, as we shall see later in the chapter. However, the ongoing trends of medical inflation and rising costs of development will exert pressure on the budgets everywhere and make access to therapies more and more of a problem. Similar arguments apply to devices – see, for example, the new robotic surgical technology described in the previous chapter.

A recent report from the well-respected Karolinska Institute in Helsinki examined the issue of cancer drug funding in some detail. The report examined the trends across the European Union and compares spending patterns in different member countries as well as summarizing worldwide issues. Globally, the cancer drugs market was valued at $34 billion in 2006, rising to $43 billion by 2008, with an annual research spend of $6–$8 billion by the pharmaceutical industry and a further $3.6 billion by the US National Cancer Institute and €1.4 billion in the EU. Around half of all the drugs in trials worldwide are cancer therapies. Within the EU, sales of cancer drugs per 100,000 population increased from less than €500,000 in 1996 to more than €2.5 million by 2007 – a six-fold increase in 10 years. Furthermore, this rise was not driven by expensive new drugs, though these are a growing strain on budgets, but mostly by increasing use of existing drugs. These two trends are illustrated in Figure 25, which shows the

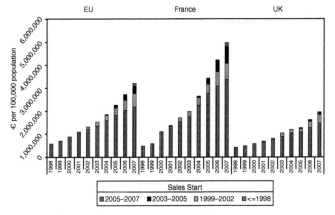

25. **Sales of cancer drugs 1996–2007 in the EU**

increase in drug spending broken down by the year in which a
drug was licensed. The figure also shows the contrast between
spending in France, where there are essentially few controls on
oncology prescribing, and the UK, where it is tightly regulated.

Why should older drugs have seen such a big increase in
expenditure? The answer lies in how drugs are licensed and then
subsequently used. If we look at figure 13 in Chapter 3 to
illustrate the breakdown of cancer therapy, we can see that
around 40% of patients develop advanced cancer at some stage,
most of whom will ultimately die from the disease. New drugs are
generally tested initially in this group of ultimately incurable
patients with limited options. In breast cancer, for example, only
a minority of patients die from the disease and hence expenditure
on a newly licensed, end-stage drug will be relatively limited.
However, if a drug works well in this group, it will often work
better in earlier patients with potentially curable disease at high
risk of relapse after their initial therapy. This group makes up
around half of the patients who end up with advanced disease.
Trials of successful end-stage drugs will thus take place in these

patients and if successful the drug will 'migrate' into the earlier disease group.

This process is well illustrated by the Herceptin (trastuzumab) story. The drug was shown to prolong survival in advanced breast cancer in 2002. From the beginning, Herceptin has attracted huge publicity. The novel nature of the treatment rapidly became known amongst breast cancer patients leading to a clamour to enter the trials. So great was the demand that a lottery for trial entry had to be set up for interested eligible patients. After the drug obtained a licence, its high price (around £30,000 per year) led to restricted access in the UK and a different sort of lottery – the post-code lottery of UK cancer funding – began for a different group of women. The subsequent highly vocal campaign by women successfully overturned the restrictions but also set a precedent for other groups seeking access to expensive therapies that still bedevils purchasing authorities in the UK in particular.

Subsequent trials in earlier disease showed in 2006 that if given to women with early high-risk disease after surgery, Herceptin reduced the chances of a disease recurrence by about half compared to previous therapies. The licence for Herceptin was thus extended to this earlier disease group the same year. Unfortunately, we cannot currently identify those who will relapse after surgery and radiotherapy. As most women in the early, high-risk group were already cured by standard therapy, the numbers eligible to receive the drug increased hugely (about four-fold in the UK) – all patients at risk have to be treated, not just those destined to relapse. Following a vocal campaign by women with the disease, the drug was made available on the NHS to all eligible patients.

How, therefore, do healthcare systems make decisions about new treatments? Suppose a new treatment costs £30,000 and improves survival by 6 months, from 12 to 18 months. What is the real cost of providing this treatment?

- £30,000
- £30,000 minus the treatment it replaces
- £30,000 minus the treatment it replaces and minus any
  consequent savings in other supportive care

There is no correct answer – it depends on who is paying for what. Answer 1 is the cost to the patient if the treatment is not reimbursed by the healthcare system. This is sometimes the case in the UK where the NHS sets limits on which drugs it will buy. The old standard of care will be covered but not the new drug. Increasingly, it is also a problem for patients in insurance-based systems where the extra drug falls outside the reimbursement package covered by the insurance. Answer 2 is the price to a hospital providing specialist care where the hospital budget per patient is fixed (as happens in hospitals in the NHS and some managed-care systems in the USA). Answer 3 is the price to the organization funding the totality of the patient's care: this may be the state via structures like the NHS or an insurance company. This then raises the further question of what exactly is included in the associated costs. For example, terminal care costs will probably be similar whenever a patient dies. However, if the survival time is longer, as in the example, they may then fall in a different financial year to the drug costs – how long must costs be deferred to count as savings? This is particularly the case with treatments which increase the cure rate, for which such costs may be postponed for many years. Again, there is no single simple answer to such questions – different healthcare systems tend to resolve these dilemmas in different ways. It is worth examining the sort of methodologies used by public health specialists and insurance companies in making these decisions on whether to fund a particular treatment.

A frequently used method is to estimate the cost per year of extra life generated by the new treatment. A correction for the overall quality of that life is often also applied. The aim is to produce a measure known as a quality adjusted life year (QALY). For example, a treatment that prolonged your life by a year but at a 50% reduction in quality would be costed as 0.5 QALY. This sounds very neat, and it allows purchasers of healthcare to compare a drug therapy that prolongs life by 3 months with a hip replacement which improves quality of life with no effect on life expectancy. For well-established treatments such as surgery and radiotherapy, patients are frequently cured, and thus this cost is spread over a large number of life years gained. Thus, although major surgery is expensive, it has a very low cost per QALY in most cases. In contrast, new drugs that prolong survival by relatively modest amounts in end-stage disease often have a very high cost/QALY, and this is where the problems start, as will be illustrated below.

An immediate problem with adjusting for quality of life is clearly apparent – how do we define how much a person's quality of life is affected? For example, Mr A leads a sedentary life and mainly enjoys watching TV for recreation, therefore an impairment which stops him running will matter very little. Mr B, however, is a keen triathlete and finds the same loss of mobility hugely distressing. Clearly, any quality adjustment is subjective and will depend on those affected. Somehow an average value must be arrived at and added to the equation.

A second problem is how to measure the gain in survival. This may seem straightforward, but often licensing trials will focus on the time taken for the disease to worsen (so-called 'time to progression' – see Chapter 4) rather than overall survival. Subsequent 'salvage' treatment may therefore improve the outcomes of the patients in the initial control arm of the trial. Endpoints for these trials are set by the regulatory authorities, such as the US Food and Drug Administration and the European Medicines Agency, and determine whether a company is granted a licence to market their product. However, just because a drug can be marketed does not mean that a healthcare system will buy it.

In order to illustrate how this process works, I will run through the recent trials carried out with a new drug in advanced kidney cancer. In the trial, patients on the placebo were deteriorating twice as quickly as those on the new drug called sorafenib. The Independent Data Monitoring Committee for the trial decided the study should be stopped on ethical grounds and all the placebo patients still alive were offered the new drug. When the overall survival times were subsequently analysed, the patients initially on the new drug lived longer than those on placebo. However, due to the salvage effect from the crossover from placebo to active drug, the survival advantage for the new drug was much smaller than would have been expected from the effect on time to progression. It is thus impossible to calculate the survival benefit of sorafenib in advanced kidney cancer as this trial can never be ethically repeated with a no-treatment arm. Any estimates for the cost per QALY for this disease are thus doubly flawed – the effect on quality of life is subjective and the true survival gain unknown. This double uncertainty paralysed the UK decision-making process for kidney cancer from 2006 to 2009.

The use of decision-making based on quality-adjusted survival has been pioneered extensively by a UK body with the somewhat Orwellian title of National Institute for Health and Clinical Excellence, usually known as NICE. This body seeks to advise the health service which treatments it should purchase on behalf of the patients and which treatments are not considered good value for money and should not be routinely funded. NICE does not consider unlicensed or experimental treatments. Some other European countries have adopted similar methodologies, but as yet the more free-market approach in the USA has shied away from such central direction. NICE will often take months or even years from the initial licence to give an opinion on a drug. In the UK, the NHS funding is split between 'purchasers' and 'providers'. Currently, the purchasers are called Primary Care Trusts (PCTs) and are tasked with making the same decisions (to buy or not to buy a particular treatment) on a local basis. At the time of writing, in 2011, this purchaser role is set to be transferred to family doctors (GPs) under forthcoming NHS reforms. The current PCTs discharge this role with varying degrees of competence and thoroughness, often simply providing the cheapest option until forced to provide a more expensive one by subsequent NICE guidance. This leads in turn to the (in)famous UK post-code lottery – as PCTs are geographically based, access to any NHS treatment is determined by the patient's address and the local PCT decision-making process. In 2008, this resulted in the highest spending PCTs allocating around £15,000 per patient for cancer care compared to around £5,000 for the lowest spending ones. In my own clinic, patients with a Birmingham post-code (a high-spend area) enjoy good access to, for example, the latest kidney cancer drugs. Conversely, most of the surrounding counties have relatively low cancer drug spends and access to the same drugs is severely restricted. As patients clearly talk to each other in the waiting room the level of frustration and anger generated can be readily imagined. We carried out an audit of survival times by post-code for our patients with advanced kidney cancer. Patients from the low-spend areas survived around 7–8 months on average, compared to around 2 years for those from the higher spending Birmingham area – a very real and worthwhile difference. In addition, patients denied access to the expensive drugs had roughly three times as many visits to hospital due to increased rates of disease complications from their untreated cancer. This state of affairs persisted for 3 years from 2006 (when the new kidney cancer drugs were first licensed) to early 2009 when NICE finally recommended that one of these drugs, sunitinib, be made available to all kidney cancer patients (though access to other recently licensed kidney cancer drugs remains heavily restricted). Clearly, the PCTs not funding these drugs would argue that they have used this money elsewhere to produce a bigger gain for a different group of patients. I am not aware, however, that there is any good evidence that poorer outcomes occur in other groups of Birmingham patients compared to their shire county neighbours as a result of lack of funds. The present UK system strikes me therefore as cumbersome, unnecessarily bureaucratic, and in many cases ill-informed. Those making the decisions, allegedly on behalf of the public, are not in any way publicly accountable for their decisions – they are not elected, for example – and often will not publicly defend them. On the other hand, in an era of rising costs, an ageing population, and shrinking budgets some form of choice must be made and thus structures like NICE will probably become more common worldwide in the future.

The proposed new UK purchasing arrangements will mean that one group, GPs, will be both purchasers and providers, with a second group, the specialist care sector in hospitals, being purely providers. It will mean GP consortia will have a financial vested interest in keeping patients out of hospitals, which may or may not be a good thing. On the other hand, they will have to justify to their own patients, in a way that the current PCTs do not, why they have chosen to refuse funding for certain treatments, as inevitably they must. It remains to be seen whether the possibility of lower management costs translates, as the government hopes, into better frontline care, as it is not immediately clear to me why GPs are the best people to decide on specialist care choices.

The cumbersome decision-making process in the UK also tends to delay uptake of new cancer drugs and reduce overall spending compared to other similar European economies. Although not formally published, it is estimated that NICE has a target spend of up to £30,000 per quality-adjusted life year gained, treatments costing more being denied funding. Other countries have less formalized methods, but appear to informally apply higher cut-off levels. Currently, the UK spends around 60% of the levels reached in countries such as France and Germany on cancer drugs as a result of this lower cut-off point. This difference seems to be particularly focused on cancer therapy as no such disparity exists in other specialisms such as cardiovascular disease or psychiatry, two other big-spend areas. This is well illustrated by the patterns of spending on sunitinib in kidney cancer since licence in 2006, with

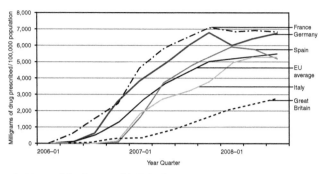

26. Usage of the drug sunitinib in the EU

the UK showing a late, slow rise in spending on the drug compared to the EU average and Italy, France, Germany, and Spain in particular (Figure 26). It cannot be a coincidence that the relatively poor cancer outcomes seen in the UK compared to our European neighbours occur in a country with a relatively low spend on cancer drugs and big disparities in spend per patient by post-code.

The future trends in spending also look challenging. There are currently 77 drugs licensed in the UK for the treatment of cancer (this ignores drugs for supportive care). Around 25 of these were licensed 1995–2005. There are an estimated 50 drugs seeking approval in the period 2007–12. Clearly, not all of these drugs will succeed in jumping the final hurdle. Furthermore, many will offer only very small gains over alternative treatment options. Some of these drugs, possibly many, will, however, offer big further gains. In addition, there will be the ongoing trend of existing new expensive drugs migrating to earlier disease settings and larger markets as illustrated for Herceptin in breast cancer. All of this will undoubtedly put further heavy financial pressure on all health economies. An interesting trend at the international conferences I attend has been discussion of these points. Until recently, this was only a topic of interest in the UK due to our relatively poor access to new drugs. Increasingly, even US speakers, with previously apparently bottomless health budgets to draw upon, have started to discuss affordability of new therapies. The healthcare reform package of Barack Obama has also put this same issue solidly on the mainstream political agenda in the USA.

There are a few trends potentially relieving pressure. Firstly, older drugs when they come off patent usually plummet in price, often by up to 95%. Secondly, if the improvement in outcome is large enough, there may be compensatory savings in other health costs, though the expenditure is now and the savings are later and may be hard to trace (and may even accrue to another healthcare provider). Thirdly, better predictors of disease behaviour may allow us to target our expensive therapies on those most likely to benefit. For example, if we knew which breast cancer patients would be cured by surgery alone (the majority), we could save a huge proportion of our adjuvant therapy drug costs. Research into such predictive biomarkers is one of the hottest areas in cancer at present for this reason. Research into new clinical trials methodologies may also help to reduce development times and thereby drug costs.

Conclusions

How these factors play out in the coming years remains to be seen, and it is likely that different solutions will emerge across the globe. Within Europe, we are likely to see the principle of universal coverage for state-of-the-art care increasingly slipping. The picture in the UK where NICE decides on affordability is likely to become more widespread as a model for decision-making, despite the problems experienced by NICE operationally. This then raises the linked issue of top-up funding, already a political hot potato in the UK. Private insurance to top up state provision may also become more the norm as the costs are much lower than for policies aimed at replacing state provision. In the USA, a major issue of partial coverage remains. Even for those with insurance, I suspect we will begin to see some attempt to limit expenditure on the most expensive cancer therapies. Outside the major Western economies, we are likely to see cancer incidence rising as life expectancy improves with economic growth. As seen in this chapter and the previous one, the best-value cancer therapies are surgery and radiotherapy, and we are likely to see a growth in these services in developing economies. The extra gain from drug therapies is relatively small, so access to these is likely to be more restricted to cheaper, older drugs, with the most expensive therapies confined to a small minority in these countries.

Chapter 6
Alternative and complementary approaches to cancer care

Research shows that at least half of cancer patients use complementary or alternative medicines in addition to conventional medicine (and one suspects that a lot of the remainder are simply not telling us). These come in many varieties and include traditional therapies used by patients from ethnic minorities. Although the terms 'complementary' and 'alternative' are sometimes used interchangeably, it is helpful to distinguish between different varieties of what may be termed to be outside mainstream medical practice. I will therefore refer to complementary medicines as those aimed at running alongside conventional therapies as a form of support. An example would be aromatherapy, which does not fundamentally conflict with the patient continuing their conventional therapy. Indeed, aromatherapy may aid compliance with treatment or reduce the need for additional medications such as laxatives or painkillers. As well as quasi-medical therapies like aromatherapy, there are treatments such as acupuncture and homeopathy that may be available both via mainstream healthcare and via other 'therapists'. Alternative medicines, on the other hand, are aimed at replacing the mainstream treatment with one that conventional medicine would regard as unproven at best and harmful at worst. In practice, it is impossible to rigidly separate treatments into one or other category, as while one patient may use a remedy alongside the conventional, another may use the same remedy in place of it – the distinction is one of intent as much as content.

There are a huge number of different alternative and complementary medicines, including homeopathy, acupuncture, dietary therapies, herbal remedies, aromatherapy, as well as techniques such as crystal therapy, visualization, and traditional therapies used by ethnic minorities. A full analysis of each of these is beyond the scope of this book, so I will try and select a few examples to make general points about how complementary and alternative treatments interact with cancer therapy. Before doing so, it is worth getting a feel for the massive extent of usage of such treatments. While countries may vary, usage in the USA is likely to be pretty typical of use in the developed world. As it is easy to quantify spending in the USA, I will give a breakdown of recent figures produced by the American National Institutes for Health. The headline figure is that 88 million Americans spent $33.9 *billion* on complementary or alternative medicines in 2007. This amounted to over 10% of all 'out of pocket' expenditure on health in the USA. In addition, a further $23 billion was spent on vitamin and mineral supplements. Given the very high medical bills faced by US citizens, it is clearly astonishing that they would spend such a sum in addition. At the 2007 exchange rate, this would have provided all healthcare for the UK population for about 6 months. These figures clearly relate to total expenditure, not money spent specifically by cancer patients; however, they do give a good feel for the extent to which these treatments are used. Similar expenditures occur in all industrialized countries. Why do citizens in all the most educated societies in the world, generally provided with healthcare which, as we have seen, keeps most of them alive into old age, shell out such huge sums on additional, mostly unproven, therapies? Clearly, in less wealthy societies, traditional remedies may be all that part of the population can afford, and thus different forces may be at play.

Before moving on to try and address this, it is worth looking at a breakdown of what the money goes on. Again, I will refer to the US figures, and clearly the split elsewhere may vary, but I believe it gives a feel of the sorts of things people want. If we understand that, it may help explain the paradox above.

The biggest category in the US report is described as 'non-vitamin, non-mineral natural products'. These are presumably herbal remedies of various sorts – as already noted, this *excludes* the expenditure of around $23 billion on vitamin supplements and minerals such as selenium. A further $4.1 billion is spent on techniques that focus on mental wellbeing with or without a component of exercise – yoga, for example. Clearly, it is debatable whether these really belong here as the individual's motivation is clear – it makes them feel good. As this clearly is a benefit in itself, I do not think further discussion is necessary. The same applies to the $0.2 billion spent on relaxation techniques.

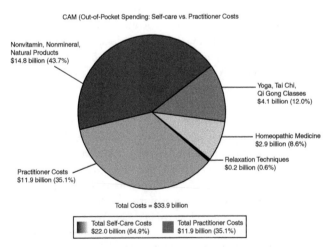

CAM (Out-of-Pocket Spending: Self-care vs. Practitioner Costs

Nonvitamin, Nonmineral, Natural Products
$14.8 billion (43.7%)

Yoga, Tai Chi, Qi Gong Classes
$4.1 billion (12.0%)

Homeopathic Medicine
$2.9 billion (8.6%)

Relaxation Techniques
$0.2 billion (0.6%)

Practitioner Costs
$11.9 billion (35.1%)

Total Costs = $33.9 billion

Total Self-Care Costs
$22.0 billion (64.9%)

Total Practitioner Costs
$11.9 billion (35.1%)

27. **Expenditure on complementary and alternative medicines in the USA, 2007**

Most of the remainder is either grouped as practitioner costs ($11.9 billion) or homeopathic medicine $2.9 billion (it's not clear whether this reflects the 'medicines' themselves or the total cost including practitioner fees). Either way, this is an astonishing sum to have been spent in a society as litigious as the USA. For a practitioner of conventional medicine, the route to a licence is long and heavily policed. Any licensed drug will have been through stringent approval procedures to demonstrate efficacy, safety, and fitness for purpose. Thus both the practitioner and products used are heavily regulated. Step outside the rules and stringent penalties apply both to practitioners and sellers of medicines and devices. Failure of either to perform to the expected standard will result in legal and often financial penalties. In conventional medicine, a drug company cannot legally sell a treatment for, say, asthma without evidence that it works a reasonable amount of the time.

For most alternative and complementary medicines, no such tests apply in most countries. Regulation is either absent or internal to the 'speciality'. No tests of efficacy apply to, for example, homeopathic medicines. Why the practitioners of these specialities are not subject to these basic rules is a mystery. Even if different rules applied, in other walks of life to charge for a good or service on the basis that it has certain properties will be subject to legal penalty if the item does not fulfil the advertised function.

The truth is that the purveyors of these remedies appear to believe that they work and their patients do likewise. Alternative and complementary therapies are therefore in reality more akin to religion than science, and this goes a long way to explaining their apparent immunity to the law, as religion itself enjoys the same degree of legal privilege in most countries. Furthermore, there is a well-known phenomenon observed in clinical trials called the 'placebo effect'. Patients in blinded trials where some are taking dummy pills called placebos will often experience the beneficial effects (and bizarrely, sometimes the minor side effects) expected from the active drug. This effect is often substantial and is in many ways highly desirable – there is clearly no risk of serious drug-related adverse events. The body is healing itself. Clearly, therefore, if the alternative 'practitioner' and the patient collude in a belief that a treatment works, it often will. Does this mean it is an honest practice? In my opinion, it does not – I believe these remedies should be subject to the same tests of efficacy as any other product, whether medicinal or not.

Furthermore, it is not the case that no harm is done by an ineffective product – it depends on how it alters the treatment of the patient. Clearly, if, say, homeopathy is used for a minor, self-limiting condition such as soft tissue injury, then no long-term harm is likely. If it is used in place of a standard therapy for cancer, AIDS, or tuberculosis (as some of its proponents advocate), then clearly deterioration can occur while the patient is forgoing some more effective therapy.

As already discussed, the gold standard way to assess any medicine, conventional or otherwise, is in a controlled trial. These are widely used to assess conventional medicines but have also been used to test complementary or alternative medicines such as homeopathic remedies as well as with techniques like acupuncture (where the control is sham acupuncture – a needle is inserted but in the 'wrong' place).

The basis of homeopathy is that 'like cures like'. Practitioners take compounds that induce a symptom, say, nausea, and then dilute the active compounds sequentially to the point when not a single molecule of the original substance remains. Proponents claim that the 'potentizing' involved in making a homeopathic remedy somehow 'imprints' the water molecules with properties that will have medicinal effects. The effects are generally held to be the reverse of the symptom induced by the agent the homeopathic pharmacy began with – hence the medicine from the example above would be used to treat nausea. For such a therapy to be effective would require a reworking of a substantial body of physics, chemistry, and tissue biology, all of which is currently lacking. Even if we concede that our knowledge of these disciplines is imperfect, it is not unreasonable to expect that there would be evidence from clinical trials of effectiveness. If there were convincing trial evidence of efficacy, clearly the underlying scientific orthodoxy would need to be re-examined to accommodate the new evidence. We therefore need to examine the clinical trial evidence for homeopathy.

A number of controlled trials with homeopathy have indeed been carried out. In 2005, the respected medical journal *The Lancet* published an article analysing the results from 110 trials of homeopathy that included a placebo. These trials were compared with 110 similar trials of conventional medicine (referred to in the homeopathy literature as allopathy, meaning 'other than the disease'). The *Lancet* article concluded there was no evidence of a coherent effect from homeopathy that could not be explained by the placebo effect. In contrast, the conventional trials were able to show effects from conventional medicines over and above the placebo in similar conditions. Homeopathy would thus seem to sit solidly in the 'alternative' category as its practitioners promote it as exactly that, an alternative to conventional medicine. With no evidence of solid benefit, this seems an irresponsible view to take, especially as homeopathy is promoted for use in all manner of diseases including potentially lethal conditions such as asthma, tuberculosis, and AIDS. This view is endorsed by bodies such as the World Health Organization (WHO) which recently issued a warning stating that the use of homeopathy to treat conditions such as tuberculosis and malaria was dangerous, and it said quite categorically that lives were being lost as a result. Hence on every level, when the 'science' of homeopathy is examined, it clearly poses problems by the yardsticks of conventional science – there is no coherent physical basis for its mode of action, nor convincing trial evidence of efficacy. Despite this lack of evidence, homeopathy is available on the NHS in the UK, and millions worldwide, including the Prince of Wales, believe in its effectiveness.

So why do so many patients use these treatments? Most people have only the most sketchy understanding of science and tend to view the claims of scientists and alternative practitioners as equally valid alternatives. This view is peculiarly limited to biology – no one wants to use 'alternative' approaches to, for example, engineering or piloting an aeroplane; they stick with the laws of aerodynamics and trained pilots. I believe that in many, if not most, cases, people are simply desperate and want to hedge their bets by backing both horses. Patients who have run out of curative conventional options often pursue these therapies and are clearly vulnerable to exploitation. Extreme varieties of these treatments often require the patient to travel to countries where regulation of such therapies is less strict than it is within, say, the USA or European Union.

Patients also frequently adopt unusual dietary approaches. Often, the underlying rationale, if there is one, will mix cause and effect. The logic underpinning these diets often runs something like this: the risk of getting a number of cancers may be increased by a lack of X in the diet (possible), therefore taking X will restore balance and treat the cancer. This leads to patients taking, for example, vitamin or mineral supplements. As a proposal, this is at least testable – we can do a trial with the supplement in question and see whether it impacts on the outcomes experienced by patients. Another common theme in anticancer diets is to pick a particular component of the diet, such as animal fat – the underlying logic being that a number of common cancers have been linked to an excess of animal fats in the diet, therefore giving up animal fats will treat the cancer (unlikely). Substituting the word 'smoking' for 'animal fats' in lung cancer illustrates the futility of this – if all you had to do to treat lung cancer was stop smoking, far fewer would die from it. Sadly, stopping smoking has very little impact on the grimly predictable outcome of most lung cancer. Similarly, evidence that these sorts of 'subtraction' diets impact cancer survival is also conspicuous by its absence. Another more recent example I have observed in patients turning up in my clinics is the claim that eating sugar is bad, as this 'fuels' the cancer. As all complex carbohydrates are digested down to sugars in the gut before being absorbed, this is highly unlikely to be a good therapy, especially as organs such as the liver and pancreas very tightly regulate sugar levels in the blood.

Despite the flawed logic and lack of evidence, patients will often adopt new diets in response to a diagnosis of cancer, frequently giving up foods enjoyed for decades to adopt a diet with alleged 'detoxification' or 'healing' properties, or adding supplements to 'boost' the body's defence mechanisms. At the extremes, both practitioners and adherents often promote these approaches with a fervour approaching the religious. Indeed, adherence to these doctrines in many ways parallels religious observance, with denial and self-sacrifice being potentially rewarded by improved wellbeing. Like religious observance, direct evidence of efficacy is not required – belief that it works is sufficient. Furthermore, failure of the technique to work can be interpreted as an indication of insufficient diligence in the application of the regime rather than an indication of lack of efficacy.

In 1990, a team of three of us (two oncologists and a psychiatrist) visited the Gerson Centre in Tijuana in Mexico. The Gerson plan is based on a curious mix of a 'detoxifying' diet (vegan, crushed fruit and vegetable juices, no added salt) and the frankly odd (regular fresh coffee enemas). Dr Max Gerson developed the diet to treat various ailments, including diabetes (he treated Albert Schweitzer) and tuberculosis. Ironically, he was driven from the USA for advocating the diet for diabetes, at the time treated with a high-fat, low-carbohydrate diet. It subsequently turned out that the 'Gerson' high-fibre, low-fat diet actually was a good treatment for diabetes, but this was only realized many years later. This does demonstrate the need to evaluate therapies in a scientific way – when this was done, it proved the value of low-fat, high-carbohydrate diets for diabetes. However, after being expelled from the USA, Gerson continued to advocate the therapy for a range of other conditions, including cancer, heart disease, and arthritis. The US National Cancer Institute carried out investigations in 1947 and 1959 to assess whether the Gerson regime had any effect on cancer outcomes, concluding both times that there was no convincing evidence of a treatment effect. Our own review of cases selected by the Centre in 1990 came to the same conclusion, which we published in the medical journal *The Lancet*. Patients at the centre undoubtedly believed they were benefiting, and in a sense, for the reasons outlined above, they were getting spin-off psychological benefits from feeling more in control of their fate. There is a flip-side to this, however, in that patients who invest a lot of energy and belief in such treatments inevitably feel that they have somehow failed when their disease worsens. This is often painful in itself, but can sometimes drive them to more extreme adherence to a regime in the mistaken belief that, if only they could adhere more perfectly, then improvement would follow.

There is a further problem with some dietary approaches like Gerson therapy. Whilst in some ways the diet (at least, without the coffee enemas) could be regarded as healthy, it may be unsuited to some types of cancer patients. For example, patients with pancreatic cancer tend to lose weight rapidly. Following a diet that will tend to bring about weight loss in healthy individuals is thus actively harmful when weight loss is part of the problem being faced. Also, as already noted, many patients tend to 'mix and match' the conventional with the alternative. Treatments such as chemotherapy can lead to digestive problems and promote weight loss. It is thus easy to see that a very high-fibre diet, relatively low in calories, may not be ideal in such circumstances. The alternative practitioner would, of course, argue that the problem here is the conventional not the alternative part of the treatment. This would be an acceptable line to run if these treatments were subject to proper scrutiny with proven efficacy. For Gerson therapy, despite 90 years of use, many published case reports, and reviews by academics, there is still not a single published clinical trial. Rather as with drugs, I feel it is for the proponents of such treatments to arrange trials, just as the drug companies have to demonstrate effectiveness to obtain a licence for their products. There may well be patients who do benefit from 'alternative' dietary approaches, but at present the evidence is lacking.

Closely linked to alterations in diet are nutritional supplements based on either vitamins and minerals or herbal mixtures (sometimes called 'nutriceuticals'). These therapies are potentially more amenable to conventional clinical evaluation than the complete lifestyle change advocated by groups such as the Gerson therapists. The simplest version of dietary supplementation is with either vitamins or minerals. Vitamins (a derivative of the compound words 'vital amines') are chemicals present in tiny amounts in foodstuffs and are essential for the body to maintain normal functions. A good example is vitamin C, derived from various fruits, particularly citrus ones. Shortage of vitamin C leads to that scourge of ancient mariners, scurvy, a condition in which wound healing is impaired, tissues become fragile and bruise and bleed easily, gums bleed, and teeth fall out – the body's so-called 'connective tissue' fails to connect things properly. Clearly, therefore, vitamin C is essential for life, but if we have sufficient, is there any benefit in taking more? The Nobel prizewinner Linus Pauling became convinced that there was benefit in so-called 'mega-doses' of the vitamin, and he vigorously advocated the practice for various ailments from the common cold to cancer (it should be noted that he got the Nobel for physics not medicine). Now here we have a readily testable hypothesis – vitamin C can be put in tablets and assessed like any other medicine. This was duly done in various settings and the answer was a resoundingly negative one – dietary supplementation of vitamin C above normal levels did not help fight cancer (or anything else). Nonetheless, hard evidence of lack of efficacy in no way prevents the alternative practitioners from continuing to promote the use of the agent, as the most cursory of online searches will confirm.

Even doing trials with simpler substances – minerals – turns out to be very difficult. For example, selenium is present in vegetables and is an essential component of tissues, being involved in the maintenance of the integrity of epithelial membranes – the lining cells of the body's various tubes and glands. It is these cells that give rise to the common cancers, and thus a lack of selenium would seem a potential candidate for a dietary top-up. Further studies demonstrated that populations with lower selenium levels had a higher risk of cancer. This prompted trials of selenium supplementation in patients with cancer, and one famous study in skin cancer showed that the patients receiving the extra selenium had a lower risk of getting a second cancer – of the prostate. The problem was, this was not what the trial was studying, but nonetheless, it was sufficient to trigger the mass consumption of selenium by men concerned about their prostates. To confirm the effect, a huge trial called SELECT was set up in the USA looking at two supplements – selenium and vitamin E. After recruiting 30,000 men, who were allocated either one or other supplement, both, or neither in a blinded fashion, the trial was stopped by the Data and Safety Monitoring Committee. By this point, the men had been followed for an average of 5 years. The Committee found that not only was there no suggestion of any benefit from either agent but, more troublingly, there was the possibility that there was a slight increase in risk of prostate cancer with selenium and, unexpectedly, the possibility of an increased risk of diabetes with vitamin E.

Even this is not necessarily the last word on the topic, however. In North America, dietary selenium levels are relatively high, hence extra may not be as useful as it would be in Europe where dietary selenium levels are lower (the difference relates to selenium levels in the soil in which vegetables are grown). In addition, selenium can be supplied as a pure chemical form or as what is known as a 'complex' linked to organic compounds more akin to the form obtained from food. Thus all we really know for sure is that the precise form of tablet used in the SELECT trial does not prevent prostate cancer in North American men. Other trials are still ongoing with both agents – for example, our own group is studying both selenium and vitamin E in men and women with early bladder cancer (also linked to lack of both in the diet) to see if supplements can prevent recurrence of the cancer.

My own opinion is that in most cases in the developed world, the levels of most vitamins and minerals will be adequately provided by most diets, particularly given the growing tendency to over-consume calories. Any effect from supplements in this setting is likely to be small, as most diets will already contain an excess over what is really needed. This is why definitive trial proof has been so difficult to obtain. As with many things in life, what starts out looking quite simple gets more complex the closer you look at it. This uncertainty, of course, fuels the market in supplements – what could be safer than taking extra 'natural' vitamins and minerals? If the men in white coats (though, of course, mostly we don't wear them any more) are not sure, why not take them just in case?

What about herbal remedies? These are, of course, attractive in the sense of being somehow more 'natural' than harsh, chemically produced pharmaceutical products. The logic is, however, intrinsically flawed – there is nothing inherently 'nice' about the natural world – watch any wildlife television show for confirmation of this. The word really has no meaning in this setting – context is everything. For example, botulism is a highly unpleasant, sometimes lethal, gut infection, but botulinum toxin is used to make people look more 'beautiful' and is certainly relatively safe as a medicinal product. The medicinal product is therefore much safer than its 'natural' source. If a herbal remedy works, it is of course because it is a drug (or more precisely, a mixture of many drugs, with varying activities and side effects).

There is also nothing magic about it being ancient (as if the length of use somehow confers an aura to it). Good examples of long-used natural remedies include witch hazel (which contains abundant salicylic acid, better known as aspirin), the opium poppy (the source of morphine and diamorphine), and foxgloves. Foxgloves are a good example of an ancient source of drugs. A brew known as 'Shropshire tea' made from foxglove leaves was used for centuries to treat the ailment known as 'dropsy' – accumulation of fluid in the lower limbs, accompanied by shortness of breath, now known to be heart failure. Then 20th-century science isolated the active ingredients – a family of chemicals named after the plant – digitalis alkaloids, of which the most commonly used is called digoxin. These drugs still form a major component of the treatment of heart failure. As far as I am aware, though, no one still uses Shropshire tea in place of digoxin.

So what about herbal cancer drugs? Well, firstly, many cancer chemotherapy drugs are indeed herbal extracts – vincristine, used to treat blood and lymphatic cancers, is derived from the periwinkle plant. The taxanes, used for many cancers including breast, prostate, and lung, are derived from the yew tree bark and leaves, and so on. Hence the study of the properties of herbs has been a major and fruitful source of some of our most potent drugs. Again, the natural source of these drugs would not make a good herbal medicine – for example, eating yew leaves is both difficult (they are very tough) and potentially fatal – the window between useful treatment effect and lethality is small.

There are examples of herbal medicines that have been tested in studies. One that I am particularly interested in is the mixture initially called PC-SPES (which stands for Prostate Cancer-*spes*, from 'hope' in Latin). This was allegedly produced from an 'ancient' Chinese herbal remedy, and marketed for 'prostate health'. Around 20 years ago, it was apparent that patients in mainline prostate cancer trials who happened also to be taking PC-SPES were deriving benefit from the herbal remedy. Despite its name, it was never tested by its makers as a cancer therapy but was licensed as a food supplement. Subsequent laboratory investigation confirmed that PC-SPES behaved like an oestrogen – technically, a phyto- (meaning plant) oestrogen. It will be recalled that oestrogens are widely used in prostate cancer therapy, and thus it is entirely plausible that PC-SPES would have anti-prostate-cancer effects. Detailed study of patients taking the mix demonstrated effects on male hormone levels and the prostate cancer marker PSA consistent with a hormonal basis for action. The clinical and chemical analyses were published in the *New England Journal of Medicine*, probably the world's premier medical journal.

This publication prompted the setting up of a trial comparing PC-SPES with a real oestrogen called stilboestrol in patients with advanced prostate cancer. The trial commenced but was stopped early due to minute levels of contamination of PC-SPES with stilboestrol. Botanic Laboratories, the manufacturers, were then shut down by the regulatory authorities in the USA, ending any possibility of completing the study. There are puzzling aspects to this story. PC-SPES had been made for years with no adverse inspections, and analysis in the original *New England Journal* article had found no contamination with stilboestrol. Furthermore, the trial, in so far as it was completed, suggested that PC-SPES was superior to stilboestrol, a result incompatible with the clinical effects being due to stilboestrol contamination, as has been suggested by some commentators.

The problem with agents such as PC-SPES is that they are only licensed as foodstuffs and hence not subject to the sorts of evaluations that a drug will have to go through. Also, the preparation is a mixture of herbal extracts, raising the question of how many components of the mix are actually required for the undoubted clinical effects seen (which included some of the known adverse effects of oestrogens such as deep vein thrombosis). The example of Shropshire tea and digoxin

- How do you assess tumour deposits in tissues such as bone or pleura (the lining around the lung) where there is no discrete lump that can be measured?

This last point is a particular problem with certain diseases such as prostate cancer that mainly affect bone. Therefore, while response to treatment remains an important test of drug activity, a second set of measures based on how long a patient takes to start getting worse – termed the 'time to progression' – is increasingly used. This has proved particularly important with the new targeted molecular therapies for diseases like renal cancer. With this disease, large masses often shrink but by less than the standard RECIST criteria. On review of the scans in these patients, it became obvious that the tumours changed in appearance, with the centre appearing to be less 'active' than before – borne out when lumps were removed and found to have dead tissue in the middle. In parallel, tumour-related symptoms often improved. For these patients, therefore, prolonged 'stable' disease becomes a very worthwhile outcome. Improved time to progression is therefore frequently used as a means of assessing activity of an agent. Finally, of course, agents can be assessed for their effect on overall survival times. This is not frequently used in phase 2 as the principal outcome for a variety of reasons, mainly time – the aim is to establish as quickly as possible which agents to take forward for phase 3 licensing trials.

Phase 3 trials

If an agent shows encouraging activity in phase 2 with acceptable toxicity, it will then proceed into phase 3 trials in which the agent is compared to the current standard of care. Where the agent is a new drug, this will generally involve the drug company discussing the trial with the regulatory organizations such as the UK Medicines and Healthcare Regulatory Agency (MHRA), European Medicines Agency (EMA), and the US Food and Drug Administration (FDA). These bodies will have an opinion as to the appropriate comparator treatment and also the outcome required illustrates the potential route of development. Unravelling this would, of course, take many years and many healthcare dollars, possibly with no patent protection to allow the company to fund these costs. We will probably therefore never know what the real active ingredients are in PC-SPES. Furthermore, although the agent looked to have clinical value, it is no longer available, though a number of similar agents (called by various names, including, in a direct reference to PC-SPES, PC-HOPE) have appeared on the market and are widely used by patients. Whether these PC-SPES clones are really the same as the original, again, we will never know. With patients taking these largely unsupervised, there is no consistent body of literature on dosing, adverse effects, and so on. In addition, as these are mixtures of herbs, even if the components by weight are the same, there is no guarantee that the actual active components will be the same in consecutive batches – anyone who has a garden will know the variation seen from year to year in the plants they grow in the same bit of ground. It is hard to see any coherent way forward given the nature of herbal remedies and the current licensing environment. Companies are unlikely to queue up to carry out trials in the future of their herbal remedies given what happened to Botanic Labs with PC-SPES. Equally, the costs of turning a herbal mix into a regular drug with potentially no patent protection seem prohibitive. The pharmaceutical industry will, of course, continue to screen herbs for useful drug properties, but the subsequent development will be aimed at a single chemical entity not a herbal brew. I suspect that these agents will be forever in a shadowy hinterland between conventional medicine and alternative practitioners. This is unfortunate, as mixed in with the large numbers of ineffective therapies such as mistletoe extracts, there will undoubtedly be agents with potentially valuable activity such as PC-SPES.

In conclusion, complementary and alternative medicines form a large and economically important activity in the health economy. However, direct evidence of benefit for most such therapies is hard to find. Furthermore, in some cases, there is good evidence of *lack* of benefit. Despite this, a large proportion of cancer patients use these treatments as adjuncts to (or in some cases, in place of) their conventional therapies. Alongside these quasi-medical interventions, there is a further arena of altered diets, supplements, and herbal remedies, again largely with little or no evidence base. Understanding usage of these treatments is important as they may confound the results of trials in cancer therapy and also may interfere with outcomes from conventional therapy, either for better (rarely, probably) or for worse.

Further reading

General considerations

There are many books about cancer on the market, mostly split between books aimed at patients and their carers and books aimed at health professionals. I do not propose to list books in the first category as they are extremely numerous, needs are personal, and also vary by country of residence. I have listed books on the technical side, and again these vary hugely – the needs of a nursing student are different from the sort of reference tome required by an oncology researcher or consultant. I have split the list into reference books and more accessible paperback works.

Detailed reference books

Vincent T. DeVita, Theodore S. Lawrence, Steven A. Rosenberg, Robert A. Weinberg, and Ronald A. DePinho, *DeVita, Hellman, and Rosenberg's Cancer: Principles and Practice of Oncology*, 2 vols, 8th edn. (Philadelphia and London: Lippincott, Williams & Wilkins, 2008). This is a very substantial textbook covering all aspects of cancer from causation to treatment of specific diseases.

Edward C. Halperin, Carlos A. Perez, and Luther W. Brady, *Perez and Brady's Principles and Practice of Radiation Oncology*, 5th edn. (Philadelphia: Lippincott, Williams & Wilkins, 2008). Another comprehensive text giving in-depth coverage of the technical background to radiotherapy and the detailed clinical application by disease.

Leslie H. Sobin, Mary K. Gospodarowicz, and Christian Wittekind, *TNM Classification of Malignant Tumours: UICC International Union Against Cancer*, 7th edn. (Chichester: Wiley-Blackwell, 2010). Cancer cases are categorized using standardized systems to allow comparison of results from different studies. This reference book gives the most widely used classification system for all the recognized groups of cancers.

Bruce Alberts, Alexander Johnson, Julian Lewis, Martin Raff, Keith Roberts, and Peter Walter, *Molecular Biology of the Cell*, 5th edn. (New York: Garland Science, 2008). Probably the definitive reference book on cell biology.

Robert A. Weinberg, *The Biology of Cancer* (New York: Garland Science, 2006). Probably the definitive text on cancer biology by one of the world's leading cancer researchers.

M. P. Curado, B. Edwards, H. R. Shin, J. Ferlay, and M. Heanue, *Cancer Incidence in Five Continents*, vol. 9 (Lyon: International Agency for Research on Cancer, 2009). Detailed reference book on patterns of cancer incidence.

More accessible shorter textbooks

Terrence Priestman, *Cancer Chemotherapy in Clinical Practice* (London: Springer, 2008).

Anthony J. Neal and Peter J. Hoskin, *Clinical Oncology: Basic Principles and Practice*, 4th edn. (London: Hodder Arnold, 2009).

Margaret Knowles and Peter Selby (eds.), *Introduction to the Cellular and Molecular Biology of Cancer*, 4th edn. (Oxford: Oxford University Press, 2005).

Betty Kirkwood and Jonathan Sterne, *Essential Medical Statistics*, 2nd edn. (Chichester: Wiley-Blackwell, 2003).

Trisha Greenhalgh, *How to Read a Paper: The Basics of Evidence-Based Medicine*, 4th edn. (Chichester: Wiley-Blackwell, 2010).

Nicholas Bosanquet and Karol Sikora, *The Economics of Cancer Care* (Cambridge: Cambridge University Press, 2010).

Other reading

Ben Goldacre, *Bad Science* (London: Harper Perennial, 2009).
    A superb exposé of the world of alternative medicine and quackery.

Websites

I have not included recommended books for patients and carers as
these are rather a personal thing. For recently diagnosed patients, or
those seeking information for relatives or other loved ones, the best
initial source is probably the Internet, as information there is likely to
be up to date and accurate, if sensible websites are used as sources.
Factors to be considered when looking at websites should include the
provider of the information. In particular, is the site selling or
supporting a viewpoint or is it independent? Many large private
hospitals, particularly in the United States, put up sites that include
information for patients but may be biased towards treatments they
themselves provide. Charities are less likely to be biased in this regard
as they should have no financial interest in treatments, but may be
slanted by fundraising needs. Government-backed sites may have
different agendas again, perhaps with a need to downplay demand for
expensive emergent therapies. It is also worth noting that treatment
patterns (and hence emphasis) will vary somewhat by country; for
example, surgery is the mainstay of therapy for advanced bladder
cancer in most countries but accounts for only about half of the
treatments in the UK. With all this in mind, it is worth consulting a
few websites to compare information. Suggested initial sites:

CancerHelp UK (www.cancerhelp.org.uk/) (accessed 21 January
2011). UK-based site supported by Cancer Research UK with
comprehensive information on all aspects of cancer and its
treatment. The site includes a listing of all trials recruiting in the
UK. The site is written in plain English for a lay audience but is
multi-layered, allowing considerable depth of information. The site
includes links to websites in other languages and countries.

The US National Cancer Institute (www.cancer.gov) (accessed
21 January 2011). Very comprehensive site with, of course, an
American perspective. Includes a large clinical trials database for
those seeking entry into a study. Also includes information in Spanish,
as well as educational materials, and sections for physicians.

Index

Index

Cancer

Index

THE HISTORY OF MEDICINE
A Very Short Introduction
William Bynum

Against the backdrop of unprecedented concern for the future of health care, this Very Short Introduction surveys the history of medicine from classical times to the present. Focusing on the key turning points in the history of Western medicine, such as the advent of hospitals and the rise of experimental medicine, Bill Bynum offers insights into medicine's past, while at the same time engaging with contemporary issues, discoveries, and controversies.

ONLINE CATALOGUE
A Very Short Introduction

Our online catalogue is designed to make it easy to find your ideal Very Short Introduction. View the entire collection by subject area, watch author videos, read sample chapters, and download reading guides.

SOCIAL MEDIA
Very Short Introduction

Join our community

www.oup.com/vsi

- Join us online at the official Very Short Introductions **Facebook** page.
- Access the thoughts and musings of our authors with our online **blog**.
- Sign up for our monthly **e-newsletter** to receive information on all new titles publishing that month.
- Browse the full range of Very Short Introductions online.
- Read **extracts** from the Introductions for free.
- Visit our library of **Reading Guides**. These guides, written by our expert authors will help you to question again, why you think what you think.
- If you are a teacher or lecturer you can order inspection copies quickly and simply via our website.